THE JOURNEY THAT CHANGED MY LIFE

FROM PROSTATE CANCER DIAGNOSIS TO COMPLEMENTARY THERAPIES AND WELLNESS

BY DAVID HEWITT & MICHELLE

Published by Purple Parrot Publishing

Printed in the United Kingdom

First Printing, 2022

ISBN: Print: 978-1-8382769-5-9

              eBook: 978-1-8382476-9-0

Purple Parrot Publishing

www.purpleparrotpublishing.co.uk

Contents

PART 1
My Journey

Introduction

I am writing this book not as an expert in any field of medicine or recovery but to share my journey, my thoughts, what I read, what I was told by the experts through from prostate cancer diagnosis (Gleason 9) to today (Autumn 2021). I have kept a diary of events and feelings throughout from September 2018 and want to relate to the reader a story of what was a difficult time, incredibly challenging and emotional at times. It is true that older men are often more reserved when it comes to talking about emotions – so read on!

I used a business technique I use with some of my clients to evaluate priorities and corrective actions called a Radar Wheel. (See later section). I found this extremely useful to rebalance my mind at the time and to focus on what was important as I slipped into a depression. Coping with mental health issues is difficult on your own and that was one major lesson learned as you will read in my story.

The book you are about to read has my story "Warts and all" straight from my diary and it describes a journey of both pain and depression to enlightenment and positivity. The cover depicts a four-leaf clover because we do all need a bit of luck on this journey and the bright light behind symbolises a light at the end of the tunnel. Not everyone will find solace in this story but if I can help one person to be more relaxed and find that "light at the end of a dark tunnel" then I would have claimed some success. I have summarised my learning points on each page.

It has been a three-year roller coaster ride for me – emotions up and down with physical and mental challenges BUT I want this story to provide hope to individual prostate sufferers because there can be an end and a positive one at that. I would like it to be an inspirational read – I want you to get the most from my experiences. Please remember this journey is MY journey of the lifestyle I lead. I didn't have excess stress factors such as a live-in partner, a career, job or financial issues.

Recently there have been several high-profile characters that have related their own prostate journey and that is great as it raises the profile and encourages guys to get their PSA tested (Prostate Specific Antigen). It's a simple blood test that provides an indication of the level of PSA in the blood. Elevated readings will require more action. I was informed that the normal level of PSA should be lower than 4.0. There is so much on the internet to help you understand the implications and actions resulting from a PSA test.

My Learning Points – keep a diary; involve close ones to you – this is not a journey you do on your own; talk about it!; insist you have a regular blood test.

My attention was directed to an article in one of the main newspapers this year and I want to relate some of the key messages to you, like understanding what and where the prostate is...

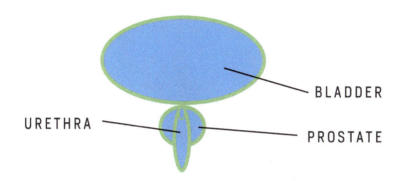

The prostate gland is about the size of a walnut and its main function is to secrete semen.

I have now realised how much misery this tiny gland can wreak in men and all because they had put off being tested. Prostate Cancer is now the most commonly diagnosed cancer.

More needs to be published on this topic to tackle men's reluctance in talking about their feelings and the treatment / testing regime they need to go through.

By the end of this book the message to all men from 40 years old is not to keep stoic and carry on but to GET TESTED before it's too late. Later in this book in part 2 there are exercises and techniques for mind and body rejuvenation to help with mental and physical anxiety.

My Learning Points – Talk about your feelings; get tested

My Story

Watching television one evening on a sunny August evening I felt so proud of the guys and girls stripping off to raise awareness of cancer. The "Full Monty" was a show arranged to raise funds and awareness of breast and prostate cancer. Needless to say, I donated a few quid that evening, it struck a chord somewhere inside me, I went to bed thinking how guys cannot recognise they have the signs.... Is it a male–thing that we just don't? Frequent toilet visits in the night and low sex drive are but two signs that are common although men think it is their age and guys get drugs such as Tadalafil and Viagra to help stabilise their libido. I dropped off to sleep.

My mother had passed away that year and I was still thinking about the times we had together and the coffee mornings we shared together, I so do miss them.

The next morning a robin appeared at my back door and would not go away, mum loved the annual visits of robins in her beautiful garden. We used to share a coffee and watch the birds in her garden. I started to talk to the robin as though mum was watching me. My thoughts turned back to the previous night and the talk of prostate cancer (I still think today that this was a sign from her telling me to get myself tested). So, later that day I decided to call the doctor. He agreed to send me to get a PSA blood test which happened that week.

The PSA (Prostate Specific Antigen) blood test is a simple unintrusive test of blood taken from the arm and results in a score of the PSA level within the blood. I was told that a reading of 4 was about the highest before an examination was required. So, on September 7th my consultant advised me that my score was 10.8 and I have cancerous cells on my prostate. I felt that a ton weight had descended upon me, I welled up inside, couldn't speak and had to drive home alone. I felt completely and utterly drained and alone – cried most of the way home. He advised I begin with scans to identify the amount of spread of the cancer – I was glad something was being done immediately and couldn't wait for the next appointment.

My Learning Points – get help from the doctor to help your sex life; keep the pressure on for appointments; regular discussion with your partner and family. Don't do this alone! GET TESTED – GET TESTED and DON'T DELAY

Six days later, on September 13th I was in the MRI scan tunnel – it took 70 minutes and to be fair was quite relaxing but a little claustrophobic. This confirmed the result of the PSA test but also that the cancer was not only contained within the prostate gland, but it had also spread just outside. To have delayed the start of this process would have been catastrophic for me. (Approximately 3000 men die every year because they leave the test too late).

It would have been Mum's birthday on September 17th – the day I had to visit the hospital again, this time for a bone scan and a biopsy. I am so glad she did not know what was happening to me (or did she?). The bone scan was negative – so no cancer in the bones. The prostate biopsy was very uncomfortable as the doctor removed 12 tissue samples from the prostate (6 on each side) via the rectum. This test was indeed to prove positive that the prostate was cancerous and had spread outside the prostate gland.

The next day – September 18th – I had a heart echocardiograph to test my heart. That proved normal, so gradually I was getting an MOT.

I clearly remember the day of the results as I attended the Rosemere Cancer Centre at Preston Hospital – I was so apprehensive and shaking that morning. My sister was visiting from Canada and wanted to come with me, and I am so glad she did, I have never felt so alone no matter who was with me. One lesson I have learned is that you need family and friends around you – a lesson I later started to ignore at my cost.

The appointment was fixed for 11am with the urology nurse who tells me the cancer is outside the prostate, so surgery is not an option. My lymph node on one side was infected. She outlines the next steps which start in 3 weeks' time, with hormone tablets then injections every 3 months. I felt a sort of relief that the hormone injection into the tummy stops the cancer spreading as it suppresses testosterone to eventually 5% and libido reduces as a result – this is something that affects men and if they are sexually active, can cause depression and self-doubt. At this time the therapy caused quite an emotional reaction as I started to fall into a very dark place. This together with the side effects of aching limbs, enlarged breasts, headaches, hot flushes and not sleeping too well at all dragged me down. I sold off 75% of my business as I was in no fit state to conduct it. The treatment was having a dramatic effect on my life, but I had to stay positive, I wanted to beat this!

My Learning Points – take someone with you to all appointments; the doctor will give you a tablet to suppress hot flushes and regular toilet breaks.

I have been into sport all my life and consider myself quite fit for my age (69). I swim and visit the gym up to 3 times a week, but the cycling had to take a back seat for now.

On September 28th I had an ultrasound on my liver, and this revealed no issues. The urology department then decided to put me on an international monitoring programme called "Stampede" where my health and wellbeing was monitored and fed into the headquarters in the USA. I was put on a daily dose of Metformin, this works to lower the amount of sugar in the blood. It affects the liver and contributes to reducing the levels of testosterone in the body. Yes, it has side effects, and these are listed on the internet, but I haven't really experienced any to date. Some common side effects are listed as stomach upsets, diarrhoea, loss of appetite, metallic taste in your mouth.

October 5th, I had my first hormone injection following the early tablets. It is repeated every 3 months. Taken in the tummy, it was a rather large needle but made me feel very emotional. I felt another wave of relief and I thought it is times like this you need a partner in your life to cuddle and talk to – I did not have that luxury. I started to push family and friends away – I felt less of a man and sort of embarrassed that I was suffering from the big C. I descended further into a dark place – one that I only experienced once before in my life after a divorce. I did not want this to go on – but I had to draw strength from somewhere to continue. At times like these you think about your family and especially the children and that brought me through this period.

A week later October 12th the hot flushes started again but this time they were quite severe and lasted weeks. I felt a bit spaced out but still continued to visit the pool to swim a couple of times a week. Exercise started to make me feel breathless and limbs ached. I started to tell myself to be more positive and that I will get through this treatment. It was now that the NHS offered a series of massage sessions which I took advantage of, and these helped with my physical and mental states – we also discussed breathing techniques to help me relax. I reviewed my diet, but my emotions were now running high – I cried every day. I got food advice from the cancer clinic, so do ask for the brochures and get help with the foods that will help you with this condition.

I decided to visit the "Walnut Group" in October – this is a group of chaps who have or have had prostate cancer. They meet on the first Wednesday each month and I started to get support through discussing my problems with like-minded people. Quite a few of the guys brought along their partners but I think in many cases they wanted to be there anyway! I could hardly speak to introduce myself to the group at my first visit... I choked and filled up – it was a very emotional hour. Since then, I found the group incredibly supportive and assisted my recovery.

My Learning Points – *keep fit – walks; some gym work and swimming weekly; don't let the depression make you push people away; join a help group; Talk it through with your partner; dealing with stress and anxiety is not easy – I felt I was drowning – breathing exercises helped me cope – take time to STOP and RELAX.*

On October 13th, the Walnut Group hosted a free PSA testing sponsored event at the local football stadium. Over 250 guys turned up and I felt a sense of achievement tinged with sadness as 10% of them returned a positive blood test. But to save one life makes all this worthwhile.

I returned to see the urology nurse and my doctor at the Rosemere Centre in Preston on October 19th – they outlined the course of treatment that was to follow – now we are moving into the unknown as my reaction to this treatment could be anything! Six sessions of chemotherapy over 18 weeks followed by 2 months rest and a scan before 37 consecutive days of radiotherapy!! This was all to kick off on October 31st plus steroid tablets and of course the hormone injections continued every three months. The emotional journey continues as my feelings were all over the place – this was to last several months. I started to feel overwhelmed.

The first chemotherapy session was quite straight forward, and I did not feel too bad during the process (Docetaxel injected into the arm) which lasted an hour. More medicines to restore white blood cells in the form of 7 days of needles, self-injected in my tummy. I went for a blood test this day – a little anxious but the result was amazing, the PSA reading had halved, reduced from 10.4 to 5.2. I started to feel the process was working – but at a cost both emotionally and physically.

The following day – November 1st I was on a high but later in the day I had an overwhelming feeling of tiredness and had to go to bed. My temperature had dropped but the next morning I was feeling ok. I wanted to get out and walk – I did 5500 steps but found I was also losing my appetite and taste buds.

The next few days my health was up and down – bombarded with drugs and injections – I lost sleep, had nose bleeds, back ache, all my limbs ached...yet I still did not want to bother anyone – pushed people away – I felt quite alone but kept telling myself that I would get through this. I telephoned the nurse at the hospital who told me the pains were partly due to white blood corpuscles regenerating after chemotherapy – I always had a good supply of strong painkillers handy (co–codamol)!!

I wanted to do more activity so on November 10th I took a bike ride only for 4 miles, but it really tired me out – my taste buds are leaving me now again.

My Learning Points – support local PSA testing events; embrace chemotherapy positively; get a healthy diet – plenty of berries and fruit/veg; I always had a supply of painkillers handy.

More chemotherapy visits in November resulted in more emotional situations for me – I can cry at the drop of a hat! Flushed face and puffy eyes – then the itching started – oh my lord it was to last 3 weeks during which time I visited A&E for some relief. I was dating someone at this time but due to the hormone injections and all the medicines I am taking my libido / performance was really suffering – I felt inadequate and continued my depression. I decided to go on the "Wagon" remove alcohol from my diet during chemotherapy. This helped!

Countdown to Christmas – still having hot flushes and aches – no side effects to metformin. Decided to restart my gym programme – treadmill / sit ups / crunches etc – this tired me but I felt quite good. I used to enjoy the gym and the swimming pool at this time – I struggled to get the energy to go, I really had to push myself, it's easier to say no! BUT when I left I felt elated. December 12th my sister accompanied me to the next doctor visit after a blood test. My PSA was down again this time to 1.27 and I felt elated. But December was a month full of hot sweats and emotional outbursts – I have shed too many tears!

A new year 2019 – started with hot flushes and emotionally drained – more chemotherapy – can't tasle my food, more fatigues and tired/aching, run down – they did tell me it would get worse, and they were not wrong. I did not want to tell everyone just how I felt – I kept my feelings to myself; this is not a good thing to do! I must keep positive, but I want to scream – no one can hear me so why not! I screamed so loud that night.

February 13th saw the sixth and final chemotherapy visit followed by more hot flushes and fatigue. I got booked in to see a psychology specialist and after a few visits it did not work so I left. The biggest challenge for me now is to get my libido back and to be able to enjoy sex again. It's going to be difficult with only 5%

testosterone in my body. Sleep patterns were all over the place and I felt like a zombie for days. Bloated and fatigued – needed to boost my immune system!

Early March the hospital sent me for a CT scan. Quite painless and no issues there.

The Walnut Group undertook a second sponsored PSA testing event – this time word had got around and 500 guys came. I enjoyed the involvement as I was organising the queues and they were long. Unfortunately, another 10% of guys were to receive letters OMG it is so common! At the end of that day my legs were aching, but I felt a sense of achievement and positivity.

My Learning Points – reduce alcohol intake; keep positive and scream if you want to – I did; Push yourself to maintain positivity.

March 25th – my third hormone injection (Zoladex) – again into the tummy - this laid me out for 2 days – joint and muscle pain, hot flushes, up all night to wee, started to feel trapped in my house. Doctor prescribed Cyproterone for the flushes but they did not work well.

Now I had 2 months off to recover before the next stage of treatments.

June 11th was the start of the radiotherapy – a one-minute dose of radiation that is 1000 times more powerful than a normal Xray - every day for 37 consecutive days (excluding weekends). The rays attack cells in the abdomen – cancer cells are destroyed, and good cells attacked but should regenerate. You lie on a bed as the "Arm" rotates around you for 2 minutes.... painless. Then I had another CT scan. Skin around the pelvic area gets dry so a good moisturiser was recommended.

As more radiotherapy visits passed, I needed to sleep a little in the afternoons just to catch up disturbed nights. Still had hot flushes – so another drug was tried – venlafaxine – I had a reaction to this so had to stop. Bowel movements were erratic.

July 31st – the 37th and final radiotherapy visit – all done!! OMG such an emotional experience. Rang the cancer bell and videoed as I left the Rosemere Unit at Preston hospital. Some family and friends were there too. I started a "Just Giving" page for Rosemere and it topped £460 within a month.

September 12th another Zoladex hormone injection – this time I had a big reaction! Rash / itching; Loss of breath, Tiredness, Constipation, Insomnia, Hot flush, Emotional tears, Dry mouth – just about everything! Lasted days and I saw the doctor.

In October, the doctor removed the hormone injection scheduled for January from my programme due to the previous reaction and my PSA was 0.8.

I had my final appointment of 2019 with the doctor on December 12th and she told me the cancer was undectable!!!!! Now it is a review and blood test every three months. It takes about 8 months to get all the medicines out of my system. In March 2020, the blood test again revealed the cancer was undetectable – I cannot understand how this is – from a Gleason score of 9 to undetectable cancer – PSA of around zero. PSA scores in June, September, December and March 2021 all came back "undetectable".

What a journey of medicines and unknowns – but I tried to remain positive most of the time! This is something that I know got me through this journey. Now with three-monthly going to six-monthly reviews I hope and pray I am through the worst.

My Learning Points – *if tired – do not fight it rest and sleep when you need to; got medicine to reduce number of bowel activities; keep positive: trying to explain to family and friends what's going on is difficult and emotional – I found having a single point-of-contact within the family group to keep everyone informed helped me.*

There is so much information / fact sheets out there that you MUST see – and if in doubt ASK!

It is true, a healthy diet does help, and we must do this even if we live alone.

Regular physical exercise, I continued to swim and light gym work, cycling and drinking 3 to 4 pints of water daily.

We don't want to increase our body mass, try and keep the weight off. I was told that a healthy weight may mean the cancer is less likely to spread and you deal better with the published side effects – which I did. There are many fact sheets on offer that give nutritional advice.

I reduced drastically my alcohol intake as advised and I was not a smoker. BUT, as always check with the cancer unit and your GP for advice.

In terms of having and maintaining a Positive Mental Attitude I found I was able to focus on the many issues and concerns and to somehow put them into priority order for me to address. I used a business concept outlined below.

My Learning Points – *get all the fact sheets from the cancer unit; they are there to help so ring them anytime; healthy diet and plenty of exercise – but not to overdo; regular doctor discussions; if in doubt either ring the GP or the cancer clinic; have a positive mental attitude and address your concerns.*

My "RADAR" Wheel to self help and a Positive Mental Attitude

This is a business technique I have crafted into a self-help tool using a collection of feelings to describe how I feel and to prioritise what I need to change (or try to).

As a qualified Engineer and Business Consultant, I used it to deal with issues and to focus on priorities. So, use this on your journey by answering honestly and openly. I hope it helps achieve satisfaction in your physical and mental states.

I had mental health issues – I went into depression, my feelings were all over the place, I was confused with what was happening to me and my body. I pushed people away, I felt less of a man, in fact I was quite a mess.

I went to counselling twice and came away with more self-worth, but I had to address so many things in my life – where was I to start? I wanted to turn negatives into positives, I needed clarity of purpose to begin this journey of recovery. I had to reach out! I had to rebalance my mindset.

Step 1

Agree with yourself the 12 topics (let us call them nodes). I used the following headings:

1. Health
2. Relaxation
3. Feelings/Emotions
4. My Partner
5. My Time
6. Family
7. My Age
8. Experiences
9. Home
10. Practical Issues
11. Finances
12. Work

These are the primary headings I needed to explore but YOU can change / add / remove headings to suit your journey.

Step 2

I "mentally sat" inside each node to identify and "brainstormed the question ". What did I mean by this heading?"

The following structure evolved over a few days – you can use this as a starter or develop your own boxes around the node or just use this model. Its function is to get you thinking just "How you are feeling" on a scale of 1 to 7 against each of the 12 where 1 is the worst and 7 is the best.

1

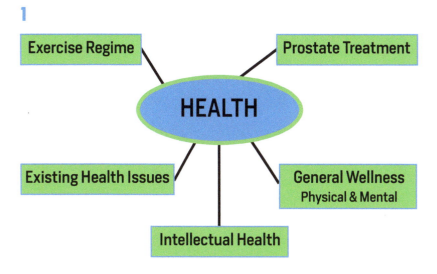

2

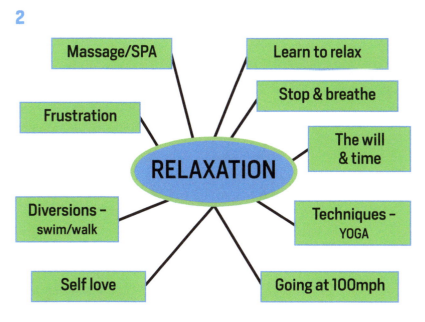

3

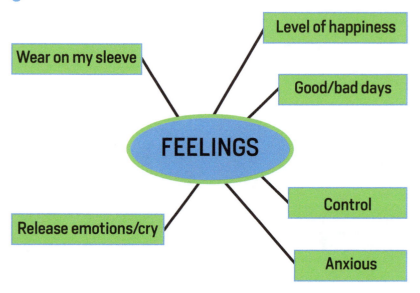

Level of happiness

Wear on my sleeve

Good/bad days

FEELINGS

Control

Release emotions/cry

Anxious

4

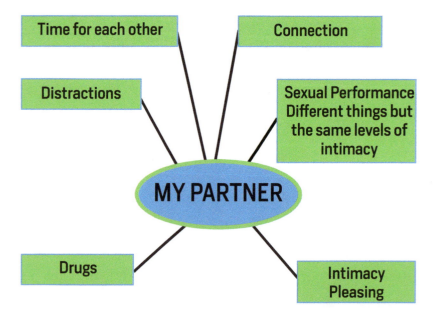

Time for each other

Connection

Distractions

Sexual Performance Different things but the same levels of intimacy

MY PARTNER

Drugs

Intimacy Pleasing

5

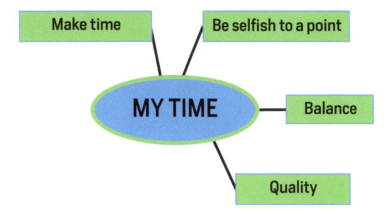

6

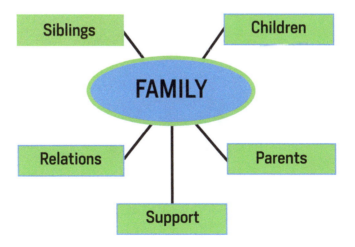

7

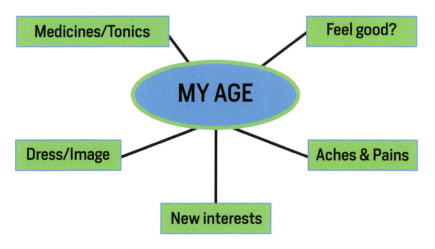

Medicines/Tonics

Feel good?

MY AGE

Dress/Image

Aches & Pains

New interests

8

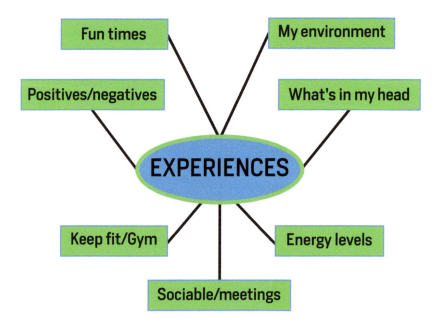

Fun times

My environment

Positives/negatives

What's in my head

EXPERIENCES

Keep fit/Gym

Energy levels

Sociable/meetings

9

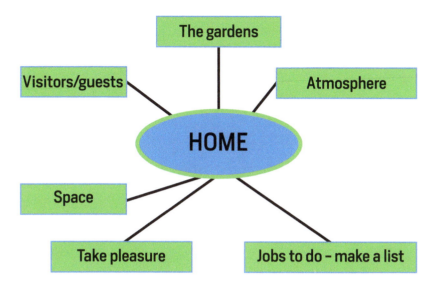

The gardens

Visitors/guests

Atmosphere

HOME

Space

Take pleasure

Jobs to do – make a list

10

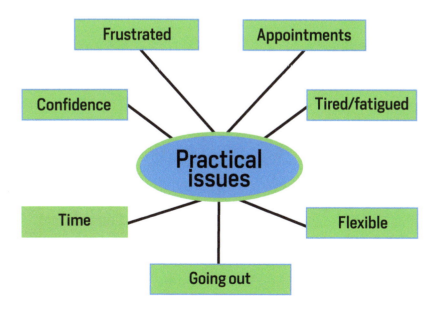

Frustrated

Appointments

Confidence

Tired/fatigued

Practical issues

Time

Flexible

Going out

11

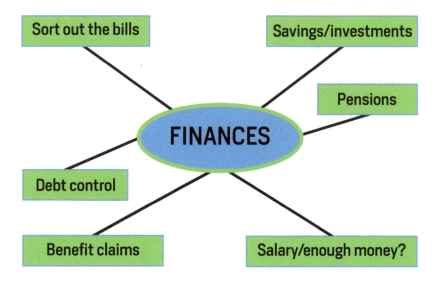

12

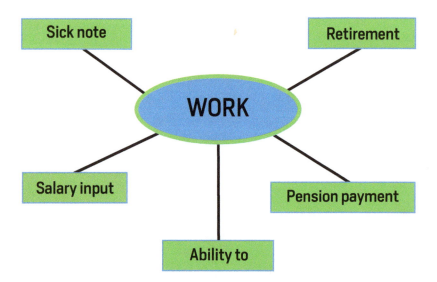

Step 3

How do you feel right now – what are your scores against the 12 categories?

Input into the chart below.... (1 to 7) where 7 is the best feeling and 1 is the worst.

The first attempt...   *Then score (1-7) monthly and add here each time*

Category	Date Month 1	Date Month 2	Date Month 3	Date Month 4
Health				
Relaxation				
Feelings				
My Partner				
My Time				
Family Issues				
My Age				
Experiences				
Home				
Practical Issues				
Finances				
Work				

Fig 1

Step 4

You now transfer the scores onto a blank RADAR Chart below (Fig 2) and join the dots to complete the picture (see example Fig 3). This illustrates the areas of positivity and the areas where there are opportunities to improve the way you feel. I used this and identified not only where I had to focus but the interdependencies between other categories and I did find relationships between the categories.

I have included the actual charts I used below:

Fig 2

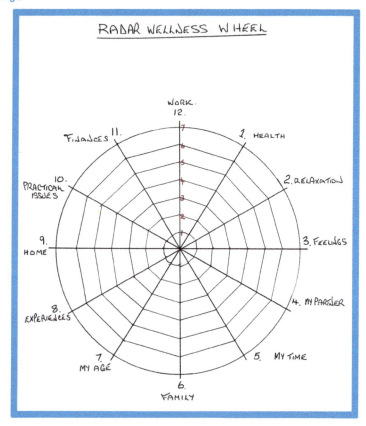

Fig 3

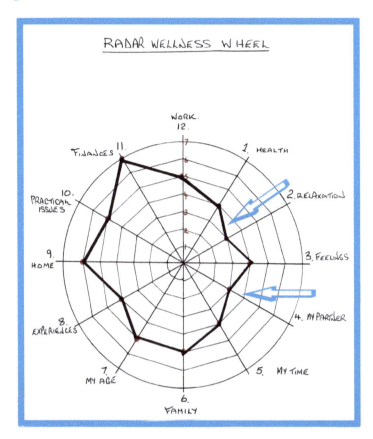

RADAR WELLNESS WHEEL

WORK.
12.

1. HEALTH

FINANCES 11.

2. RELAXATION

10.
PRACTICAL
ISSUES

3. FEELINGS

9.
HOME

4. MY PARTNER

8.
EXPERIENCES

5. MY TIME

7.
MY AGE

6.
FAMILY

Lines that are nearest the centre are obviously the low scores – but these are the areas of opportunity to address first – this process prioritises our actions.

In this example the areas to address first are in the first and second quarter of the wheel – interdependencies are the other categories around the low scores.

Fig 3 above (having experienced this range of scores) my personal conclusions would include: –

a) Relaxation techniques (and we discuss later in this publication)

b) Relate relaxation to the feelings you and your partner have.

c) Look and see if there is a relationship with your health & relaxation.

d) Check on medicines with doctors' advice.

e) Find more time to not only be with your partner but also for yourself.

These were my thoughts – you must identify what you need to do from the summary of your information above.

By taking actions – ANY ACTIONS for the above – you can review and rescore a month later – update the chart (Fig1) and redraw on Fig 2. These will monitor progress – but it also: –

• gave me goals to achieve.

• priorities to address.

• involved other people close to me.

• gave me a purpose.

• illustrated a barometer to use month to month to see progress.

• after several months I could see and feel improvements to my mental state.

I found this self–help process easy and simple to use in order to visualise and prioritise the important and urgent areas to focus and work on. Visualisation techniques are used across industry

– this is just an adaption of one technique that I found to be so useful.

Towards the end of my treatment, I found the side effects were still bothering me. I decided to book a week in Tenerife to cheer myself up and hopefully feel better – at least to get some sun. I had become accustomed to the island to just fly in and flop on a sunbed and recharge the batteries. I had usually booked in for regular treatment during my stay to see Michelle (a Holistic Therapist). I have grown to know and respect the work she does and to know that there will be some benefit by seeing her. I read somewhere that holistic therapies focus on boosting relaxation and reducing stress associated with living with and surviving prostate cancer – something I needed on this visit.

I booked my appointment with Michelle as usual on my arrival – it was nice to see her again as I had come to know her over the years – she sensed something as soon as I walked into the treatment room. I remember she asked about my health and true to form over the past 12 months I broke down to tell her my story. The treatment included Reiki and gentle reflexology. Afterwards I really felt at peace, calm and relaxed. I had finally let my guard down – it felt good as though a burden had been lifted and I walked out into the sunshine.

I decided to continue with complementary therapies on my return home. I attended several massage sessions through the NHS and found that it helped immensely. I can personally recommend that, for me it worked to relax and relieve muscle pain and increase psychological well-being.

About a month after my return, I was tested and the PSA reading was zero! I felt elated!

I thought about telling my story – I wanted to help people, to present my perspective, my recovery, the things I did to improve my recovery. So, I decided to share this story which is so important to me.

I asked Michelle if she could help in any way with this book – her contribution would prove to be invaluable.

Please read on – Part 2 – this is next...

PART 2
The Wellness Journey

Introduction

Before I introduce myself and the wellness journey to you in Part 2, I would like to take this opportunity to thank David for sharing his journey with me. Without his determination, positivity, patience, willingness to learn, belief and trust, our contribution towards prostate health and prostate cancer awareness would never have happened. His motivation to always want to improve the situation, that giving up was not an option for him and to choose to have a positive mindset through adversity and fatigue, for me, is truly an example for all.

David's story has a happy ending, but it did not come without some blood, sweat and tears. My intention in sharing with you a programme which I put together for David to refer to and use during the second part of his journey and beyond, is to help others to also have easily accessible information on complementary therapies which may help them too through adverse times. The information provided also helps improve prostate health and wellness in general.

For many there are days when you may feel like doing nothing, ill or not. My hope is that within the pages of this book you may learn that there is always a little something you can do, however small, to help you feel just that bit better.

I hope that in sharing this information it may also encourage others to embark on their own personal wellness journeys and I wish you all the best of luck too, because as David said, "We could all do with a bit of luck".

Warm wishes
Michelle.

Wellness for Mind and Body

Prostate Health and Prostate Cancer – A Holistic Approach

During David's stay in Tenerife, we took the time to sit down and discuss the issues which had been most difficult for him to cope with during his journey, this enabled me to understand which aspects of my natural health knowledge would be useful and helpful to him. I offered to put together a personal programme for him to try over the following months, which he willingly accepted to do. The various subjects we covered are included within part 2.

This Wellness journey is based on my knowledge from training in holistic therapies, Traditional Chinese medicine and Hatha Yoga principles. Holistic means treating the body as a whole. I have tried to incorporate as many health aspects as possible including internal organs, joints, energy balance, mind, body and soul. By addressing the body as a whole in a holistic way, it sets the fertile ground for healing and wellbeing to occur. (For more info visit: www.mholistictherapies.com).

David found that this was quite a different approach than he was used to. Although many people may know how to keep fit or follow basic diet guidelines, much is often missing in looking after the body as a whole. This holistic approach helped him to understand the importance of mind body connection to feel balanced which is fundamental for overall wellbeing.

David was encountering on his prostate cancer journey particular issues such as anxiety, stress, sleep disturbance, aches and pains to name a few. My intention was to introduce David to self-help techniques, based on ancient wisdom to help him address these problems and to add a feeling of being a little more in control.

I discovered during the journey how difficult it can be to encourage a man to want to stop and relax for a bit without a good reason, so I hope that you will find within the following pages the good reasons as to why this is so important for health, particularly during times of illness and recovery!

David has told me that since he started this wellness journey, his attitude has completely changed and he now paces himself more consciously during activities and his use of energy within everyday life. He says he feels more balanced, less fatigued and happier. The results and benefits he has found since he started the programme have definitely had an undeniable positive impact on his overall health and wellbeing.

The Wellness Journey

The Wellness journey offers information on natural therapies, easy self-help techniques and skills to incorporate into your daily life. It covers various categories which are all as important as each other to improve overall health and wellbeing. The information provided was offered to David for use during his treatment, recovery and afterwards.

The information has been divided into sections to use at your convenience for physical movement and mind / body relaxation techniques. I have tried to condense the information into a practical guide and starting point for many. Each of the categories has been broken down into bite size chunks with the idea that you can pick and choose what is helpful to you at any given time. Every body and every person is unique with different levels of energy and health. It is important to choose what works for you and that you find enjoyable too!

- BREATHING EXERCISES – For stress and anxiety.
- DAILY MOVEMENT – Use it or lose it.
- RELAXATION – Refresh and restore the body.
- MINDFULNESS and MEDITATION – Relax the mind.
- ENERGY MANAGEMENT – Recharge.
- DIET – To fuel the system.

The wellness journey, as outlined in the following sections, was designed to be gentle and restorative as it is important to conserve energy for healing. It gives the body an opportunity to rebalance body systems, refresh and reset.

It is important to understand that when we use energy (output), it must be replaced by input (relaxation). Rest and sleep are also an important part of the healing process as they give the body an opportunity to restore and repair.

It is recommended to do something every day, as it is the consistency that counts. You can start small and work up, doing as little or as much as you feel like on the day. In general, a minimum of 10 to 15 minutes is valuable in balancing body dysfunction, however even if you only manage 5 minutes it helps make a difference to your wellness.

By dedicating time for ourselves daily we are giving our bodies a chance to do their best. It helps us to be stronger, reduce recovery time, improve the immune the system and lift our mood. It's worth a try..

Ultimately, wellness is the ability to listen to one's own body and mind, understand your own needs and take the actions to meet them. It is also important to remember that an integral part of any wellness programme includes regular health check-ups, creating healthy habits and a positive attitude to help you along the way ☺

Keep Calm and Do Yoga

* A Body and Mind in Balance Is Key to Your Health and Wellbeing *

Why practice Yoga?

Yoga uses breathing exercises, meditation, relaxation techniques and poses to stretch and flex different muscle groups. Yoga helps to reduce stress, calm the mind and connect mind and body.

By caring for our bodies as a whole and addressing each of the following aspects, the mind body connection is balanced and wellbeing is enhanced.

Physical – muscles, joints, ligaments, bones, blood circulation, internal organs, digestion etc. The fluid movements and poses also help to correct posture and increase energy.

Mental – calms the mind to help cope better with adversities.

Emotional – helps lift mood and enhance wellbeing.

Spiritual – connection to self, others and the environment around us.

> *Yoga techniques may help men deal with the side effects of prostate cancer therapy.*

Yoga for Prostate Health and General Wellness

Yoga teaches us how to transform negative stress to positive.

Positive stress can motivate an individual to develop creativity and strive for achievement. Negative stress can lead to ill health, depression and inertia.

To reduce stress the body and mind must be treated as one. The tension associated with stress is stored mainly in the muscles, diaphragm and the nervous system. If these areas are relaxed, stress is reduced. There are specific yoga poses for an enlarged prostate to relax and release tension, some of these have been included in the daily warm up section of this book.

Unlike any other form of exercise, yoga gently rejuvenates the body internally and externally whilst releasing tension and stress. A yoga practice has many beneficial effects which affect every part of your wellbeing.

This natural approach can help enhance prostate health and general wellness.

It is considered that the five principles of yoga which are breathwork, relaxation, meditation, diet and exercise, should be addressed daily in some way for good health. These principles are covered within this book in which you will find some user–friendly guidelines to help make this possible. Should you find they are beneficial, it could also be helpful to share these principles with others you know so that they may also reap the wellness benefits within their own lives ☺

Yoga for Men

The Best Workout You're Not Doing

Yoga makes you stronger in new ways by targeting aspects of fitness that traditional exercise does not. Not only are the original roots of Yoga very much in the male domain but there are also a whole host of very real powerful benefits of YOGA FOR MEN.

Doing an activity such as yoga may also be helpful towards improving prostate health. It can aid in the prevention and possible reduced risk of prostate enlargement, along with the problems it can cause.

Benefits:

- Improved Mobility And Posture:
  −Helps counter the effect of sitting in a chair all day
  −Improves core strength which benefits balance and posture. The exercises also help to strengthen pelvic floor muscles.

- Enhanced Strength And Flexibility:
  The asanas (postures) help build muscle which supports the joints, they also help build bone strength. Flexing and gentle movement adds for healthy joints and tendons.

- Weight Control And Gut Health:
  Deep breathing, twisting and bending help massage the internal organs which benefits digestion and the immune system, metabolism is also increased. The hormone cortisol, which forces the body to hold on to belly fat, is reduced with deep abdominal breathing exercises.

- More Productive:
  Increases mental resilience, helps deal better with stress, be less vulnerable to burnout and improves mood.

- Beats Stress:
  Contributes to heart health and reduction of blood pressure, which increases body's ability to respond to stress in a positive way.

- Not Competitive:
  Instead of focussing on external competition, yoga forces you to turn inwards and focus on your own personal growth.

- Improved Sleep Quality:
  Yoga calms the body and mind. It is perfect for stress relief as it relaxes the nervous system and helps decrease anxiety.

A Typical Yoga Class Based on Traditional Hatha Yoga

When I first mentioned the concept of yoga to David and how it could help him, he went to try a few classes to see what it was all about. The outcome was that he found, at that particular stage of his journey, that it was an effort to go and came back feeling tired and achy. This is where we decided it could be a good idea to put a wellness programme in place to allow him to regularly do something of his choice every day from the comfort of home and depending on his energy levels on any given day and until such time in the future when he may feel to participate in yoga classes.

There are many different styles of yoga, my recommendation is to start with gentle Hatha yoga. Yoga retreats, workshops and classes provide an atmosphere and environment that is ideal to learn and practice the poses, relaxation, meditation, positive thinking and proper breathing techniques before starting to practice them at home.

Below you will find some useful information on yoga classes, tips and what to expect.

What it involves:

- Pranayama:
  —Practice of breath regulation exercises for physical and mental wellness.

- Warm up:
  —Concentrates on warming up the joints to prepare for the poses.

- Asanas:
  —Practice of body posture, pose or position. Helps improve posture, flexibility, strength and balance.

- Relaxation:
  —Extremely therapeutic, gives the body a chance to refresh and restore itself whilst lying down.

• Meditation/visualisation:
–Classes may end with a short period of guided meditation or visualisation to help silence the mind. This is followed with some quiet time before gently incorporating ourselves back into daily life.

A yoga session in general takes approximately 60 to 90 minutes. You can attend group classes or see a private teacher for instruction. You should tell your teacher about any medical problems before you begin, they can adapt the poses to suit your needs. A good yoga teacher will be able to show you the poses which are particularly beneficial for prostate health and make sure you move through the class at a pace which is right for you. You should never force or feel at any time you are creating any type of stress in your body. You should come out of the class feeling relaxed and refreshed.

It is important to take things gently at first to minimise the risk of injury and be sure during the practice to tell your teacher if any posture is painful for you. It is recommended to allow at least 2 hours after eating before doing yoga and drink plenty of water after every class.

If you are following treatment, it is important to join a gentle class to begin with so that you don't come out feeling worn out!

The Importance of Breathwork

Breathing is immediately connected to all levels of our bodies and has to be seriously considered when we talk about health.

Breathing practices can help reduce emotional exhaustion, improve your mood, help reduce burnout and provide a natural intervention for stress, depression, anxiety, aches and pains.

When under stress our emotions are heightened and breathing becomes quick and shallow, which creates anxiety and muscles tighten. We can feel overwhelmed, fearful or out of control. Breathing and our emotions are intimately tied together.

Stress in the right quantities does not lead to ill health. However, when the pressures of life exceed a certain limit (which varies from person to person) anxiety or depression can result.

Correct breathing techniques can help reduce stress and anxiety by calming the nervous system and help improve sleep.

Controlled deep breathing engages your rest and repair state that starts the relaxation response. This is a deep rest for your body that allows it to heal.

Breathwork exercises help remove toxins (carbon dioxide) and increase oxygen levels in the blood. They also help strengthen the immune system.

It is scientifically proven that nasal breathing improves oxygenation by 20% and delivers purer air to the lungs, compared with mouth breathing, which is shown to increase respiratory stress, fatigue and increased chance of infections.

The regular practice of breathwork (5–10 minutes a day) offers a multitude of physical, emotional and mental health benefits. There are different types of breathing exercises, some to calm the nervous system down and others to energise. By practicing controlled breathing and saving your breath you can also help to save some of your energy.

Breathwork is a valuable life skill to master helping to keep mind and body in balance. Used as a strategy in stressful situations it instantly helps to calm, feel more centred and in control. It is fundamental to all relaxation, anxiety and stress reducing techniques. It is quite amazing how a simple breath controlled in the right way can make all the difference to your health and wellbeing.

Note:

- *It is not recommended to do breathwork exercises if suffering from a cough/cold.*
- *Breathwork exercises must always be done in a seated or lying down position, never standing up.*
- *When doing the breathwork exercises, find a quiet space where you will not be disturbed.*
- *It is preferred to practice on an empty stomach.*

Yogic Breathwork Techniques

In this section you will find examples of yoga breathing techniques which I selected for David to use depending on his feeling and to help to be calm and relaxed.

In doing these exercises, we found it also helped to get in touch with emotions by rebalancing them and helped in releasing by letting go any negative ones ☺.

In Yoga, the practice of breath control is called Pranayama. It is considered that this ancient art is key to achieving balance and healing in one's life.

Pranayama

Benefits for physical and emotional health:

- Can help reduce anxiety, depression and stress.
- Can help cope with panic attacks.
- Helps cope with aches and pains.
- Helps you to rebalance body systems and relax.
- Can help improve sleep quality.
- Can help with insomnia.
- Can help decrease fatigue.
- Boosts the immune system.
- Helps reduce high blood pressure.
- Helps improve lung function.
- Develops breath control.

- Helps improve digestive system function.

- Helps increase oxygen levels in blood.

- Enhances cognitive brain function, performance and focus.

- Promotes sense of inner calm.

- Increases mindfulness.

Yogic breathwork emphasises attention to breath, often taking long deep inhalations and exhalations.

- *INHALATION – is breathing in the new, energy, fresh air (oxygen) into the body.*

- *EXHALATION – is the removal of the old, stale air, toxins (carbon dioxide) from the system.*

- *When the breath becomes calm, it also helps us to focus and still the mind.*

Steady the Breath to Steady the Mind

Safety and Precautions:

- *Stop the practice immediately if you feel any adverse effects, such as shortness of breath, dizziness, feeling lightheaded or nauseous. You should not feel any discomfort or pain during your practice.*

- *Talk to your doctor before starting practice if you are unsure or have a medical condition such as asthma, COPD, or any other lung or heart concern.*

- *Please consult with your GP if you are unsure.*

Breathwork Exercises

Three Part Breath - Calming and Grounding.

The 3-part breath begins in the lower belly, rises to the lower rib cage and finally moves into the upper chest and throat. It descends from collar bone to ribs to belly. It teaches you to breathe fully and completely.

A calm nervous system encourages good health and ensures a more controlled mind. This type of breathwork is one of the most calming, grounding breathing exercises that you can do and helps overcome shallow breathing. This technique is taught to relieve stress and even to address panic attacks. You can use it throughout the day whenever you are feeling any tension. Even two or three breaths will have a positive effect.

This breathing exercise really works to focus your attention on the present moment, to get in tune with the sensations of your physical body and helps when experiencing pain. It is also extremely beneficial in helping to improve sleep quality and insomnia when done just before going to sleep.

Benefits:

- Nourishing, calming, relaxing.
- Can help improve sleep quality.
- Can help with relief of panic attacks.
- Helps calm nervous system.
- Can help when experiencing pain.
- Can help lower/stabilise blood pressure.
- Strengthens respiratory muscles.
- Massages abdominal organs, improves lymphatic drainage and circulation.

Instructions:

1. Sit in a comfortable position, feet flat on the floor, lengthen your spine. (Can also be lying down).

2. Relax your face and body, breath gently and naturally through your nose.

3. Place your right hand over your belly and your left hand over your chest. Close your eyes.

4. Begin to focus your awareness on your breath as it moves in and out through your nose.

5. Inhale into your belly, slowly and deeply. Feel your belly expand.

6. Exhale completely pressing abdomen gently to help expel air and feel belly deflate.

7. As you continue with the inhalations from your belly, then increase breath to feel the expansion of your ribs and then to the base of your throat.

8. As you exhale, relax the upper chest, feel the ribs contract next and lastly deflate belly. Continue at your own pace (from point 7) slowly, starting with the belly then moving upwards eventually coming to let the three parts of the breath happen smoothly without pausing as you repeat each round.

- *Each breath should flow naturally without tension.*
- *Repeat 5 to 10 rounds of this breath.*
- *Be careful never to force the breath or breathe too deeply.*
- *It is important for your lungs to feel comfortably full, but not strained.*

The 3-part breath is often done while seated in a comfortable position, however it is particularly beneficial and relaxing for prostate cancer patients to do it whilst *lying on your back*. When you are lying down, you can really feel the breath moving through your body as it makes contact with the floor/ mat/ bed. You could also *add a gentle rocking motion of the pelvis*, *this helps to release tension in the pelvic area*. With each inhalation gently rock the pelvis forwards and with each exhalation gently rock back so your back is flat on the floor, gently drawing navel to spine as you fully exhale.

Cooling Breath - Beat the Heat!

I have found with my clients that this type of breathwork can be effective in cooling the body when experiencing hot flushes to help decrease severity. It can also be helpful to use when feeling overheated on a hot day or if you are stressed/angry.

Benefits:

- Cooling and soothing for mind and body.
- Helps to balance excess heat in the body, helps regulate body temperature.
- Helps reduce agitation and irritation.
- Helps reduce high blood pressure.
- Adds moisture to the system.
- Helps reduce fatigue.
- Helps reduce excess bile which causes heartburn.
- Helps controls hunger and helps quench thirst.

Instructions:

1. Sit in a comfortable position. Lengthen your spine.
2. Rest your hands on your knees. Close your eyes. Exhale completely.
3. Make a tight 'O' shape with your mouth.
4. Roll your tongue into a 'U' shape and project it out. *
5. Inhale slowly through your mouth filling your belly for the count of 4. Feel breath move into mouth and back of throat.
6. Close mouth, hold for 2 counts, exhale through your nose for the count of 6, deflating belly.
7. Pause, relax, repeat from points 3 – 6. Continue gently for up to 3 minutes.

* *(if you are unable to curl your tongue, simply flatten tongue, purse lips to make a small 'O' shape and breathe through mouth).*

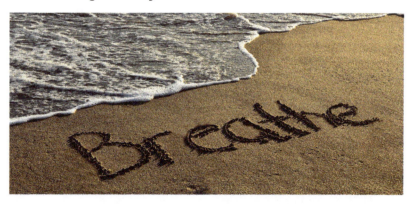

Alternate Nostril Breathing – Reset and Refresh.

This type of breathwork is often used in mindfulness and relaxation methods to help calm the body and mind and has wide reaching benefits.

Benefits:

- Promotes overall wellbeing.
- Relaxes body and mind.
- Reduces stress and anxiety.
- Cleanses and strengthens the entire respiratory system.
- Expels stale air and waste products from lungs.
- Improves oxygen absorption in the cells.
- Balances left and right hemispheres of brain.
- Balances parasympathetic nervous system.
- Can help to balance hormones

Instructions:

Basic technique:

1. Sit in a comfortable position. Lengthen your spine.
2. Place your left hand on your left knee.
3. Lift your right hand up towards your nose, bend first and second fingers towards palm.
4. Exhale completely and then use your right thumb to close your right nostril.

5. Inhale fully through your left nostril for the count of 4, then close left nostril with 3rd finger.

6. Release thumb from right nostril and exhale completely through this side for the count of 8.

7. Inhale fully through the right nostril for the count of 4, then close this side with thumb.

8. Release 3rd finger from left nostril, exhale completely through this side for the count of 8.

- *This is one cycle.*

- *All breaths are deep belly breaths. A belly breath means that as you inhale your belly expands outwards and as you exhale the belly deflates completely as you pull it back towards the spine.*

- *Continue your next rounds from points 5 – 8 for a few minutes. Always complete the practice by finishing with an exhale on the left-hand side.*

- *Take a moment for your breath to return to normal.*

Once you get the hang of this basic breathwork technique, you can include an additional relaxation technique to enhance the practice.

- As you continue with this breathing exercise, now close your eyes. Notice the flow of your breath as it moves from one nostril to the other.

- Continue with the left right nostril breathing taking a moment to bring your attention to the area just between the brows. Soften the brow and face and feel your body start to relax.

- On your final exhalation, place your hands in a comfortable position and continue to focus with the eyes closed on the area just above your brow, scan your body as you continue to breathe slowly, relax and let go of any remaining tension.

- Take a moment to enjoy the peaceful sensation before gently opening your eyes.

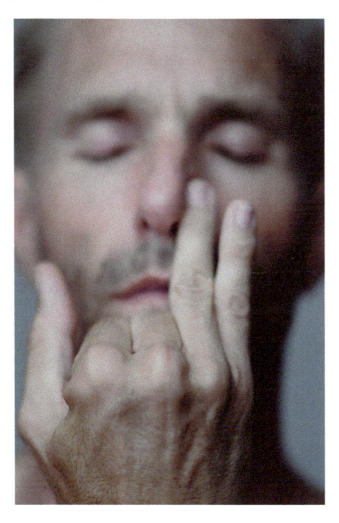

"Quickies" – Basic Breathing Techniques.

Below you can find breathing techniques which are easy to use quickly in everyday situations to help with better stress management.

Quick Calmer – 4-fold breath

Need to calm down fast? Try this quick exercise. It is also known as box breathing.

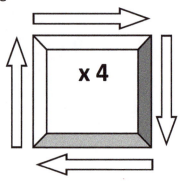

Instructions:

1. Sit down and align yourself into a straight posture, feet hip distance apart. Gently exhale all your breath out.

2. Gently inhale through nose for count of 4 expanding belly.

3. Hold for 4 counts.

4. Gently exhale through mouth for 4 counts deflating belly.

5. Hold for 4 counts.

6. Repeat gently for 4 rounds.

The counting of the breath helps to focus and quieten the mind.

Beat the Butterflies – Abdominal Breathing

Breathe deeply when you become afraid or tired? When anxious we tend to take rapid shallow breaths that come directly from the chest, which makes pressure rise. This exercise helps bring pressure down by concentrating on belly breaths.

Instructions:

1. Sit down and align yourself into a straight posture. Keep shoulders relaxed.

2. Take a slow deep breath into the belly, feel it expand without forcing it, inhaling through the nose.

3. Without pausing, or holding your breath, gently deflate belly by exhaling through your mouth, keep jaw relaxed.

4. Repeat for a few minutes until you feel calmer.

Summary:

Breathwork can really be helpful not only for those on their prostate cancer journey, but also for maintaining a healthy balance in everyday life in general.

It has also been found helpful for libido as it helps decrease stress and anxiety.

Activity and Rest

Life Balance

The Importance of Balance in Our Everyday Lives.

When I went to study in China, I was fascinated by the way the people worked, rested and exercised. In the early morning large numbers of people go to the parks to practice energy balance exercises, known as Qigong or Tai Chi. Some would walk, some would dance, some would sing, some would hum, all of which have health benefits which are described later ☺.

It was all part of their daily health practice.

Later, in the middle of the day, it is common for people to take a short nap after their lunch. Workers asleep in their carts, office workers put their heads down at their desk and elderly doze on roadside seats. It is considered that digestion requires energy and this energy should be replenished. Although this is very different from the western world, I did learn the importance of energy output <> energy input. i.e., to learn to STOP and give our bodies the chance to replenish and recharge.

Many westerners lead lifestyles which are out of balance. Some are far too overactive and some are far too underactive. It is considered best to balance our work, relaxation, exercise and sleep within each 24-hour cycle. It is also suggested that we should regularly remind ourselves of the 70% rule when exercising, this means that you would regularly move at 70% of your total capacity at any given time to prevent burn out.

It is considered the hours before midnight give the most nourishing sleep. Sleep is important to strengthen organs and replenish energy reserves.

All areas must be balanced. If we take care of ourselves by eating properly, getting enough rest and exercise and practicing techniques that release tension from our bodies, then our immune system is greatly improved and our resistance is fortified.

We can only withstand a certain amount of stress. Each person has a different threshold and each must determine for himself or herself how much is too much. When you create an inner awareness of what's going on inside you, both emotionally and physically, you discover your optimum balance of activity and rest.

Life Balance During Illness

I introduced this concept to David both during his treatment and recovery. I explained that everything had to be kept well balanced to aid healing, from diet to exercise, energy saving and relaxation to rest and sleep. In the following pages you can find some of the activities and suggestions which I gave to him, which he still uses to this day for his general wellbeing and health maintenance.

Make Finding Your Balance Part of Your Daily Life Routine

Exercise

Daily Exercise

Stretching and aerobic exercise are the two most important types of exercise to practice daily for health maintenance. Gentle stretching (5 minutes twice a day) keeps your muscles and joints loose. Aerobic exercise (20–30 minutes) swimming, cycling, running, brisk walking develops muscle tone, stimulates deep breathing, sweating and increases blood circulation.

Deep breathing exercises are also important. They are known to be holistically, the most gentle and effective methods known for purifying and revitalizing the body. If your breathing is shallow, your body's vital systems are not functioning at their optimal levels. When you breathe deeply however, the respiratory system can fully oxygenate and help rejuvenate the body.

Exercise naturally regulates and balances your whole system. When you don't exercise, your metabolism can become sluggish and the tendency to get depressed or overeat increases.

External Exercise

External exercise is any exercise which focuses primarily on strengthening the body. They include running, cycling, swimming, Pilates, martial arts or playing other sports.

Internal Exercise

Internal exercises are different. They focus on movements which activate the inside of our bodies and their organs and tend to be gentler than external exercises. Tai Chi, Qigong and

Yoga come under this heading. The focus of our concentration is within ourselves, rather than what is going on around us and the movements are made in a mindful way. The result of doing these internal exercises is that we develop internal strength and become calmer and healthier from within.

A holistic approach to health understands that internal and external exercises are beneficial for our health and the need for both.

Note:

Whilst gentle aerobic exercise such as walking and swimming is recommended for everyone, men with prostate cancer should avoid prolonged cycling because of the pressure the seat puts on the perineal area, which is between the scrotum and the anus. The selection of exercises you will find on the following pages will help in maintaining a healthy prostate.

Exercises for Prostate Health

These exercises are combined with the aim to enhance prostate health and wellness, or to help with an enlarged prostate in a natural way. They can be used as a preventative measure, or during and after prostate treatments.

• Daily warm ups
  The **movement** section gets energy and blood flowing in and around all parts of the body and the organs to nourish them. The gentle **stretching** exercises are designed to release any tension in the pelvic area and relaxing muscles for the correct function of the prostate. When the area is too tense urine has difficulty in passing.

- Balancing exercises
  Core strength helps to support and stabilise spine and pelvis, balance and posture. The balancing exercises help with this.

- Qigong exercises
  These movements help to recharge e*nergy and vitality*.

- Kegel exercises
  Although relax and release is important, a balance must also be found in having **strengthened pelvic floor muscles** to support the bladder and bowel. These exercises can also help with *incontinence*, providing better bladder control and urine flow. They can also improve *sexual function* in some men.

Daily Kegels for Prostate Health

The first thing to know is which are the muscles you need to be contracting and relaxing! Kegels are subtle and require some concentration and practice to get them right. Perseverance and daily practice are the key to success ☺.

Precautions:
- Make sure you are hydrated before doing these exercises.
- Do not overdo Kegel exercises.
- Do not do these exercises if you have a catheter fitted.

When to do Kegels:
- Daily.
- If you are going to have surgery for prostate cancer, or if you have an enlarged prostate.
- After treatment for prostate cancer to help with problems of getting or keeping an erection.

Instructions:

- One way to find your pelvic floor muscles is to stop and start your urine stream whilst you pee. The muscles you use to stop your urine flow are your pelvic floor muscles. To pull in your pelvic floor, think of pulling in and lifting up your genitals. Learn to isolate your pelvic floor muscles, if your stomach moves, then you are using those muscles too!

- Start by tightening and holding your pelvic floor muscles in for 5 seconds then slowly relax your pelvic muscles between each squeeze.

This is one Kegel exercise. You should plan to do 10 to 20 Kegel exercises up to 3 times a day.

Make sure to keep all other muscles relaxed whilst you do this exercise. Do not tighten the muscles in your stomach, buttocks or thighs. Do not hold your breath or push down.

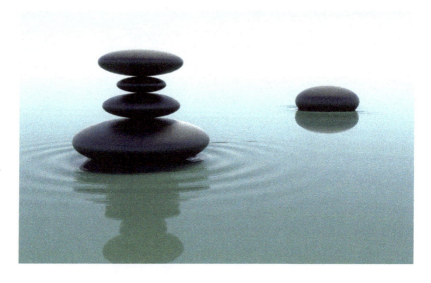

Daily Warm Up Sequences

The daily warm up movements consist of a series of movements which effectively aid in freeing stiffness and toxins from joints and muscles, helps to relieve tension in the pelvic area, aids blood flow to extremities and aids digestion. They only take a few minutes and can be practised any time.

Depending on energy levels or movement ability, the daily warm up sequences may be practiced from either lying down, seated or standing positions.

I personally enjoy creating body awareness whilst doing each move by being mindful of each action, feeling the movement, then gently relaxing and releasing any tension as I go along. I also like to practice slow belly breathing throughout the sequence which helps to balance the nervous system and find that by the end of even a short warm up, I feel much improved than before I started ☺. I consider this time as important 'me time' and a necessary part of self-care for wellness.

The warmups can be done during the day when you feel like it (although not just before going to bed). I find I get greatest benefit in the morning time as it wakes your system up and gives a healthy mental attitude to continue the day with...

These mobility moves can also be practised after sitting or standing for long periods of time to loosen everything up and get blood circulating again, rather than it stagnating.

Let's Get Started ☺

Before starting any of the daily movements, begin with a few minutes of gentle breathing to relax you into the present moment. This enables your mind to be focused to take more care as to how you are really doing each move and to observe as to how your body is feeling and responding. This is known as mindful activity and is a wonderful way to learn how to listen to your body whilst keeping everything working! Mindfulness itself is used as a therapeutic technique. It is a mental state achieved by focusing one's awareness on the present moment, while calmly acknowledging and accepting one's feelings, thoughts and bodily sensations.

By taking a moment to be mindful and concentrate on the moves, it helps us to feel more centred and in control, then as you connect with your breath you start to feel calmer. Take a moment to relax between each move before asking your body to go on to the next one, be aware of how your body feels and acknowledge what each movement does for you.

Being mindful is a mental asset that helps significantly in regulating mood and emotions.

Stretch and Flex – activating all joints

It is considered important to exercise joints to keep them healthy. By exercising your joints more synovial fluid is produced which is necessary for them to work freely and easily. This fluid also helps in keeping bones slightly apart, helps protect cartilage coverings from wear and tear and helps absorb shocks in the joints.

Standing Sequence - total time approximately 7-10 minutes

1. Stand comfortably feet shoulder width apart, arms gently by your sides and spine straight. Feet remain shoulder width apart throughout sequence.

2. Take a relaxing breath and on the exhale, roll shoulders back and down so they are comfortable.

3. Start to relax your body and turn your concentration to the flow of your breath. Let it flow gently and naturally.

4. *Qigong twists* – (see instructions in following Qigong section on *page 89*). Do this exercise for approximately 1-3 minutes.

5. *Lower back rub* – Gently rub kidney area with knuckles.

6. *Spine stretch* – With a full belly breath, stretch arms over head as far as possible, clasp fingers together and pull upwards so your body is fully extended. Hold for a moment feeling the stretch up to the sky. Relax.

7. *Shoulder rolls* – Continue with belly breaths and place fingers onto shoulders. Keep tailbone tucked in. Gently circle shoulders 6-8 times backwards, feeling the chest lifting and opening. Repeat in a forward direction 6-8 times, feel the stretch across your back.

8. *Pendulum* – Gently lower chin to chest. Roll chin slowly from shoulder to shoulder like a pendulum side to side to loosen neck 6 times. Take care once finished when raising head back up to be slow and gentle.

9. *Finger stretch* – Interlock fingers, push palms away from you to gently stretch fingers, release and relax.

10. **Wrist circles** – Lift arms in front of body to 90 degrees and do wrist circles 6 – 8 times in each direction.

11. **Hip circles** – Place hands on hips. Circle only hips, rest of body remains still, 3 times in each direction making large circles.

12. **Pelvic tilts/rocks** – These are great for both relaxing pelvis and working pelvic floor muscles. Hands on hips, knees softly bent, gently rock pelvis forwards on an exhale. Engage pelvic floor muscles by pulling in and lifting genitals upwards, bring tummy inwards towards spine as you tuck your tailbone in. Hold for a second, then relax and release muscles as you gently rock pelvis backwards on an inhale.

    Repeat move 6–8 times. (For more information on pelvic floor exercises see the Kegel exercise section).

13. **Opening knee circles** – Place hands on bent knees. Gently make outward knee circles 3 –6 times, then inward knee circles 3–6 times (take care if you have any knee issues).

For the next 3 exercises, should your balance not be too good, then you could use a wall or chair for support.

14. ***Ankle circles** – Engage tummy muscles, lift foot. Do ankle circles in both directions, 6 to 8 times each way .Repeat on other side.

15. ***Toe stretches** – Raise heel off ground (as though wearing high heels)! Bend toes and gently push into ground to feel the stretch. Repeat on other side.

16. ***Toe roll*** – (only if no broken toes)! Place foot into 'high heel' position. Gently roll toes over to feel stretch on topside of foot. Repeat on the other side.

17. **Forward fold** – Standing feet shoulder width apart and knees slightly bent, exhale as you slowly let your body fold forwards as far as you can go, letting arms, neck and head hang loosely. Rest for a moment feeling the stretch before gently rolling back up to standing position. Roll shoulders back and relax. This fold helps to relieve pelvic tension.

18. ***Mountain pose*** – Finish off by standing straight with arms by side, body relaxed, take a moment to concentrate on 3 deep belly breaths filling up your body with fresh oxygen and then relaxing, releasing and letting go on the exhale.

If you have time and wish to continue with a moment of further relaxation to allow your body to refresh and restore then continue with the next relax and release section.

Relax and Release – time approximately 5-10 minutes.

- Relax - Finish off by sitting or lying down. Place arms by your sides, palms facing upwards. Observe your gentle natural breath flow.

- Release – Body scan – Take your attention to your toes, notice how they feel, notice any tension you may find and release. Follow with your attention slowly to every part of your body all the way up to your face and to the top of your head, relaxing releasing and softening the area as you let go. Be sure to cover all areas, from the toes to top and bottom of feet, ankles, calves, shins, knees, thighs, groin, lower back, hips, abdomen, chest, shoulders, arms, hands, palms, fingers, spine, back of neck, jaw, ears, cheeks, lips, tongue, teeth, nose, ears, eyes, forehead, top of head.

Stay for the time that feels good to you for the relaxation. When you finish, sit quietly for a moment before getting up. If lying down, gently roll over onto your right-hand side before slowly getting up.

Lying Down Sequence – total time approximately 8 minutes.

1. Start by *lying down* comfortably, preferably on a mat, on the floor, palms facing upwards.
    (If lying flat is uncomfortable you could pop a small pillow under knees for support, or gently bend knees with feet flat on floor).

2. Start to *relax* your body and turn your concentration to the flow of your breath. Let it flow gently and naturally.

3. *Extension* – Stretch arms over head as far as possible and stretch legs and toes as far as possible, so your body is fully extended for 3 breaths.
    Relax arms by sides– feel the effect.

4. *Ankle circle* – Engage tummy muscles, lift leg to 90 degrees. Do ankle circles in both directions, 6 to 8 times each way. Repeat on other side.

5. *Wrist circles* – Lift arms to 90 degrees and do wrist circles 6– 8 times in each direction.

6. *Finger stretch* – Interlock fingers, push palms up to the sky, gently feel the stretch in all your fingers, release and relax.

7. *Lower back massage* – Slowly bring knees up to chest, place hands on knees and do gentle circles, 3 times in each direction. Feel the gentle massage effect on lower back area. Finish with a **bear hug** by interlocking fingers together on knees and on an exhale, raise chin to knees gently. Release and relax.
(The 'bear hug' helps aid digestive organs and excess wind).

8. *Hip circles* –Bring knees to chest, put hands on knees. Keep feet together and let knees gently fall open to the sides. Make full circles with knees in an outwards direction 3 times and an inwards direction 3 times.

9. *Butterfly bounce* – Place feet back on floor, knees together, chin to chest. Gently let knees fall apart, keeping soles of feet together. Place hands on belly and gently bounce knees so you can feel the hips slowly opening (this helps to **stretch and release inner thighs and groin area**). Relax and continue with belly breaths for about 30 seconds until you can feel the area loosening up. Finish by gently bringing knees back together and place feet flat on floor, hip distance apart.

10. *Bridge raise* – Place arms by sides, palms facing down, keep feet flat on floor. Contract glutes and core muscles. Gently push through heels raising bottom off floor vertebrae by vertebrae into a bridge position. Hold for a moment before gently releasing and relaxing

slowly downwards towards floor, vertebrae by vertebrae. Take a breath before repeating raise a couple more times. (Avoid this exercise if you have an injury, or are recovering from surgery involving back, abdomen, pelvis, hip or knee joints and ankles).

11. **Pelvic rocks** – Place hands palms facing down by your sides, feet hip distance apart. Let lower back sink flat onto mat, exhale and engage pelvic floor muscles by pulling in and lifting upwards the genitals and hold for a second. Now release and gently let your pelvis rock forwards so that there is a little arch under your lower back, inhale and fill belly as you move. Repeat the gentle rocking motion for up to 8 – 10 rounds. (For more info on pelvic floor muscles see the Kegel exercise section).

12. **Spinal twists** – Place arms out to the sides forming a 'T' shape, palms facing down. Bring feet together and gently let both knees drop slowly towards the floor from side to side in your own time to loosen spine.

13. **Relax** – Finish off by sliding feet down slowly so legs are straight and you are once again lying flat on your mat. Place arms by your sides palms facing upwards. Observe your gentle natural breath flow.

For some added relaxation you can continue for a moment by doing the body scan.

Release – Body scan – Take your attention to your toes, notice how they feel, notice any tension you may find and release. Follow with your attention slowly to every part of your body all the way up to your face and to the top of your head, relaxing releasing and softening the area as you let go.

Stay for the amount of time that feels good to you for the relaxation. When you finish, gently roll over onto your right-hand side and sit for a moment before slowing getting up off the floor.

Balancing Exercises

By doing the balancing exercises both balance and physical coordination is enhanced. A good sense of balance is important to keep us steadier on our feet. In yoga, balancing exercises are also found to be very helpful in relieving stress and reducing inner tension.

Apart from the physical balancing exercises you can also do brain balancing exercises which help to balance the left and right hemispheres and control the amount of information received to avoid 'overload'. This is necessary for overall good brain health and function.

This special set of exercises can be done any time, every day of the week, or just a few times a week.

I personally find that doing the balancing exercises regularly helps to keep me strong, calm, focused and centred.

Why developing balance is important:

- To help avoid injury.

- Increases strength and stability.

- Improves communication between muscles and the brain (neuromuscular communication)

- Develops mental and physical stability.

- Promotes stillness in your mind.

- Develops greater body awareness.

- Improves posture.

- Helps strengthen core muscles. (These deep stabilising muscles include the pelvic floor, the innermost layer of the abdominal muscles and the muscles on either side of your spine. Together these muscles completely encircle your spine from front to back like a corset. Strong core muscles also help protect your lower back).

Tips:
- *For beginners it is recommended to have a chair, or nearby wall as a support to lean on, if necessary, until you gradually build up your strength to hold your balance.*
- *Start easy and work your way up as you go.*

Let's Get Started ☺

Foot Raises

Benefits:

- Strengthens core, hips and lower extremities.

- Improves distribution of body weight and posture.

Instructions:

1. Stand comfortably, arms gently by your sides and spine straight.

2. Take a relaxing breath and on the exhale, roll shoulders back and down so they are comfortable.

3. Gently tuck tailbone under and engage core muscles.

4. Gently raise one foot off the ground to a comfortable height so you are balancing on one leg. Count to ten.

5. Gently replace foot to ground.

6. Take a relaxing breath before repeating on other side.

- *As you progress, try to maintain the one-legged stance for longer periods of time.*
- *Remember to stay as straight as possible and not to lean to one side.*
- *Keep back straight and core engaged.*

Tree Pose

This extremely grounding yoga pose is an excellent way to improve concentration and focus as well as clearing the mind, as to do it, you really have to be focused on what you are doing in that present moment!

Benefits:

- Improves posture.
- Improves overall balance.

- Increases hip mobility and strength in the lower body.

- Tones and stretches inner thighs, calves, ankles, groin.

- Helps strengthen core muscles.

- Brings emotional and mental balance.

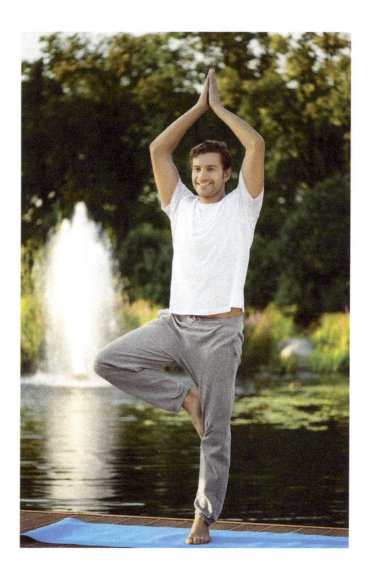

Instructions:

1. Stand comfortably feet shoulder width apart, arms gently by your sides and spine straight.

2. Take a relaxing breath, roll shoulders back and down so they are comfortable.

3. Shift your weight onto left leg, draw right knee up and in towards your chest.

4. Turn right knee out and place sole of foot onto the ankle of your straightened leg.

5. Slowly reach your arms out and then up with an inhale. Bring your palms to touch overhead.

6. Gaze at one point ahead of you. Hold the pose and take slow deep breaths.

7. When you are ready, slowly release your arms and leg down with an exhale.

8. Change sides and repeat.

> **Modification:**
> As your balance improves, gradually move sole of foot to calf, then to inner thigh. Never place foot onto knee.

Brain Balancing Exercises!

Balance and coordination exercises help to keep us physically and mentally nimble by using our ability to balance and coordinate muscle activity. Whilst many physical games and sports require this type of coordination, for prostate cancer patients we wish to recharge our energies, rather than expend. This is why yoga, Tai Chi and Qigong type practices are more favourable for improving your balance and coordination when fatigued, as they are more energy saving.

For brain synchronization (the balancing of the left and right sides of the brain) we practice in yoga the left right nostril breathing exercise, which can be found in the breathwork section of this book. This breathing exercise helps improve the communication of thoughts and responses. This results in better performance and improves mental and emotional health.

Another brain coordination exercise is to clean your teeth with the opposite hand. By asking our brains to do something different, we must think and concentrate in a different way which is said to strengthen neural pathways.

Energy Management/Qigong

About Qigong

Qigong is a form of ancient Chinese health exercise. "Qi" means 'Vital Energy', and "Gong" means 'Cultivation'.

The aim of Qigong is to promote the movement of energy, known as Qi in the body. In our youth we tend to have limitless energy but as we age our reserves tend to dwindle. Qigong can help us to focus on recharging our inner batteries with vitality.

All Qigong styles focus on cultivating and increasing the supply and flow of energy throughout the body. By increasing this energy flow, it is believed to promote longevity and induce calm mental and emotional states. Doing Qigong requires little expenditure which is very handy if you don't feel like doing much but still would like to do something.

Qigong can roughly be divided into three main categories: Martial Qigong, Spiritual Qigong and Medical Qigong. Qigong uses a wide variety of movement styles, including shaking, stretching, self-massage, coiling and swinging motions, as well as slow flowing movements and challenging static postures. All Qigong techniques emphasise the use of a focused mind, good posture and relaxation.

It is said that where our mind goes our energy flows, so when we practice Qigong the idea is that our mind is fully involved. When the mind is directed inwards and connected with how our body feels in that particular moment we can become aware of how it feels energetically. By noticing the areas of weakness, tension, contraction or even numbness and encouraging a better flow of energy to those areas, we encourage the body to rejuvenate.

Most medical Qigong exercises are carried out by slowing down, softening and becoming relaxed to allow energy to smoothly circulate around the body. In studies it has been said to show that practicing Qigong and Tai-chi may help reduce pain, depression, fatigue and improve life quality for cancer patients.

Qigong is easy to learn and enjoyable to do. Even a few minutes practice can have an invigorating and rejuvenating effect.

The following Qigong exercises were integrated into David's programme to help recharge his energy and vitality. The exercises can be practiced either separately or put together to form a sequence.

For a *'quick'* energy boost you could do the *twist* and *shake it* all out Qigong style!

Qigong Stretch - Rebalance energies and relax mind.

Benefits:

This exercise is a complete stretch. It strengthens all the internal organs and stretches the spine to help back problems. Practicing it daily will strengthen breathing and help create a smooth flow of Qi throughout the body.

Instructions:

1. Stand relaxed with feet shoulder width apart, knees slightly bent and feet facing forwards. Place hands just below navel, palms facing downwards and with fingers pointing towards each other.

2. Breathe in, imagining that you are taking vital, pure Qi into your body. At the same time bring your hands outwards and upwards in front of the body so that the palms are held high above the head facing upwards, keeping back straight.

3. Breathe out and at the same time lower the hands out to the sides while bending the knees slightly. Imagine that you are clearing any stale or impure Qi through the fingers.

4. Bring hands back to the starting position.

5. Repeat this exercise at least 10 times every day. The benefits will be felt from it only if it is performed on a regular basis.

Qigong Twists - Activate energy and healthy spine.

It is considered that keeping your body and spine flexible contributes enormously to overall general health maintenance, particularly as we age.

Just this movement alone is also a great stress relief technique and great to incorporate into a work break, as it counteracts the tension created by prolonged sitting. Excess sitting can contribute to digestive disorders and anaemia to name a few, so this is an easy way to get some energy circulating around your body. This exercise is quite stimulating so also a good one to do in the morning to get going!

> • *Do not practice this exercise if you have a back injury, slipped disk or have had any recent surgery.*
>
> • *Always make sure you are hydrated before performing any sort of exercise. If you feel dizzy stop immediately and sit down.*

Benefits:

• Energises immune system.

• Relieves tight muscles.

• Loosens and relaxes neck, shoulders, back, arms.

• Massages spine and internal organs.

• Relaxes the nervous system.

• Helps improve digestion.

• Helps improve poor circulation.

Instructions:

Try to find a balance between your spine being both long yet relaxed. Good postural alignment helps the flow of Qi, but the excess tension of perfectionism tends to constrict it.

1. Stand straight, feet shoulder width apart, knees soft, tail tucked in to lengthen spine, arms hanging heavy by your sides.

2. Take a few breaths gently in through nose and out through mouth.

3. Start to swing arms loosely around body, try to engage core muscles as you go.

4. As swing gets looser, start to twist gently from waist side to side, keep head in line with belly button.

5. Gently amplify twist as far round as feels comfortable.

6. Let arms flop and gently wrap around body with each move letting your hands gently tap body around hip and waist area.

7. Continue focusing on the move for a few minutes for as long as feels comfortable then gradually slow down swing until you stop.

8. Finish off by gently rubbing kidney area with knuckles.

9. Relax for a moment.

Shake it out – Unblock and release.

This is one of the simplest Qigong exercises

Benefits:

* Helps clear stress and transform it into vitality.
* Gentle increase of blood circulation helps detoxify th body.
* Helps keep joints flexible.
* Relaxes and warms all muscles, organs, joints and fascia.
* Can help support function of kidneys and adrenals.

Instructions:

1. Try to relax and let your whole body go completely floppy.
2. Place feet shoulder width apart, softly bend knees, sink feet into ground.
3. Smile! This helps create positive energy.
4. Gently start a bouncing motion.
5. Shake your all limbs loosely to release tension.
6. Breathe in through the nose and out through the mouth long and deep.
7. Continue for as long as you feel comfortable, gradually slow down to a minimum bounce before finally stopping. Take a moment to relax and notice how your body feels.

Energy Savers / Tips

By doing the best for our health in a preventative way, we are giving our bodies the best chance to do their best. Here are a few ideas to consider.

Rest and Sleep

The time given to rest and sleep is time given to our bodies to restore and heal. Any body system which is over stimulated will eventually under function!

During the night our Qi withdraws inside us and nourishes our organs. If we don't get enough sleep and rest we will not be replenishing our energy and in time this will draw on our reserves and we deplete ourselves. About a third of our life is spent sleeping. To enable us to get the greatest health benefits from sleeping it is important that we sleep in a good posture and are relaxed. A traditional posture to allow Qi to flow freely is to lie on our right-hand side with the top leg bent and the other leg straight. The right hand can be placed under the head or the pillow and the left-hand rests on the thigh. In this position the heart is high up so does not get constricted and the liver, which the Chinese say "stores blood', is lower down and hence receives more blood.

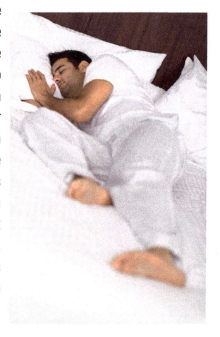

There is nothing worse than tossing and turning and finding it difficult to sleep. It is recommended to first 'relax the heart'. This means that we should try to go to bed not excited, nervous or over stimulated. To sleep better here are some suggestions:

1. Cultivate going to bed at a regular time each night, even if you don't immediately fall asleep.

2. Cut out stimulants such as coffee and tea.

3. Follow the 3hr rule. Leave 3hrs for digestion of food before going to bed.

4. Avoid stimulating activities for at least 1hr before going to bed, including watching TV. All electronic devices, exciting books etc.

5. Do a relaxation breathing exercise.

Energy Drainers:

- Conflict.
- Heavy meals, alcohol.
- Mobile phones, screen time, social media.
- Rushing.

Energy Savers:

- Remove yourself from stressful situations wherever possible, your body will thank you for the energy saved.
- Digestion requires a lot of energy, by choosing healthy options and avoiding cold drinks you save energy.
- Build the extra time in to slow down. Be aware of time management.

- Avoid overload. Know what your stress limit and energy output limit is. Learn to balance it out using energy balancing techniques and exercises.

Energy Raisers:

- Walk in nature.
- Relaxation time.

Relaxation, Meditation and Chakras

The Importance of Relaxation for Your Health

Relaxation – Definition: When the body and mind are free from tension and anxiety.

Relaxation is not only about peace of mind or practicing a hobby or activities we enjoy, it is an essential process that decreases the effects of stress on your mind and body. Your mind has a direct effect on your mood, immune system and health in general. By calming the mind, we give the message to our physical, mental, emotional and energetic body that it is time to restore and reset. The only time the mind tends to rest is when we are asleep, or during periods of deep relaxation.

Rest is when we cease activity and motion, both mental and physical, complete rest is considered to be when we sleep. Sleep is necessary to rest your mind and repair the body. Rest and relaxation are crucial to optimum functioning and to avoid burn out.

By using relaxation techniques, you can help to release tension in both the mind and body for a period of time. This can help you to enjoy a better quality of life, especially if you have an illness. Relaxation also improves our ability to cope better with adversity.

Deep relaxation helps us to calm down whilst we are awake and gives the body chance to replenish its energy supplies by slowing it down. It also creates a space to restore the normal functioning level of the body. In general, after taking a break for relaxation, the mind and body are more rested and work better for whatever task is at hand, including healing ☺.

There are many ways to relax so take yourself temporarily out of the game for a while to stop, replenish, release and let go. Your body and mind will thank you for it.

Relaxation techniques

In general relaxation techniques involve refocusing your attention on something calming and increasing awareness of your body. There are many techniques available for relaxation, meditation and mindfulness. It is a good idea to try a few to see which ones work best for you. It really doesn't matter which one you choose, what matters is that you try to practice relaxation regularly, just 10 minutes a day can make a difference to your health. Free apps are available online with a varied selection of meditations and soothing online recordings to choose from. Many find that with the mindfulness practices, the more you do them, the more natural it becomes.

Benefits:

- Reducing muscle tension.
- Improving mood and concentration.
- Lowering fatigue.
- Improved sleep quality.
- Reducing anger and frustration.
- Reducing stress hormones.
- The heart, arteries and blood vessels are given a chance to restore and the mind is given time to relax and calm down.

Relax Your Thoughts – Relax Your Mind

Examples of deep relaxation techniques

All the below techniques help to calm the mind and give the body a deep rest so it can heal itself from stress. They may be practiced either seated comfortably or lying down, whichever you find most relaxing. Make sure you are in a quiet space where you will not be disturbed for full benefit.

Breath focus. In this simple, powerful technique, you take long, slow, deep breaths (also known as abdominal or belly breathing). As you breathe, you gently disengage your mind from distracting thoughts and sensations by concentrating on the inflow and outflow of the breath.

Body scan. This technique blends breath focus with progressive muscle relaxation. After a few minutes of deep breathing, you focus on one part of the body or group of muscles at a time and mentally release any physical tension you feel there.

You could start by concentrating on your toes and moving up through all the different areas of the body to your face and top of your head. A body scan can help boost your awareness of the mind-body connection.

Guided imagery. For this technique, you use your imagination to conjure up soothing scenes, places, or experiences in your mind to help you relax and focus. You imagine using all your senses, vision, taste, sound, smell, touch. Your body can become more calm and relaxed in response to calming, peaceful and pleasant thoughts

Guided meditation. This is focused purely on the mental state, without the addition of whole body senses, it helps the mind find peace and balance.

Mantra meditations. For this technique, you silently repeat a short prayer or phrase while practicing breath focus. This technique helps the mind to stop wandering as brain is given something to focus on. Here is an easy one to start with, it is simple, effective and easy to learn.

Instructions:

1. Sit comfortably, close your eyes.

2. Begin with belly breaths, breathing deeply into the lower abdomen. Take a moment to observe the inflow and outflow of your breath.

3. On the next inhalation take a slow deep breath through your nose while thinking the words "BREATHE IN, RELAX ".

4. Then exhale slowly through your nose while thinking the words "BREATHE OUT, LET GO".

5. Continue to allow your breathing to flow easily whilst silently repeating the words with each inflow and outflow of breath. Feel your body start to soften and relax with each inhalation and release and let go of all tension with each exhalation.

6. Whenever your attention starts to drift to thoughts in your mind, sounds in your environment or sensations in your body, gently return to your breath silently repeating the words.

7. You can continue for as long as feels comfortable, starting with 5 to 10 minutes and working up to more, if you wish, depending on the day.

8. When you have finished, sit quietly for a moment with eyes closed before moving.

Visualization. This involves picturing positive images, ideas, symbols or using affirmations and mantras to help calm the mind whilst the body is in a relaxed state.

Visualization Quickie. This is a great way to instantly lift your mood. When energy is down think of something that you enjoy, something that makes you feel good. Close your eyes for a moment and imagine the place, smell, taste and feel the emotion it creates as you enjoy the experience it in your mind. When you are done you will notice you have created more of a feel-good factor which makes your mood feel lighter ☺.

Chakras – Rainbow Visualization Technique

Some colours are associated with relaxation and can be a helpful way to clear the mind of tension and allow meditation to start.

I introduced David to the concept of the "Chakra" system for energetic rebalancing which he enjoyed.

Chakras form the basis of an ancient approach to healing and balancing our physical, mental, emotional and spiritual selves and are considered a subtle part of our energy system. These energetic 'nerve' centres are described as spinning wheels of energy located within the spinal column. There are 7 chakras, and each has a corresponding colour that follows the colours of the rainbow: Red, orange, yellow, green, blue, indigo and violet. They are considered important energy centres to help us feel well balanced and calm, which in turn affects our overall sense of wellbeing.

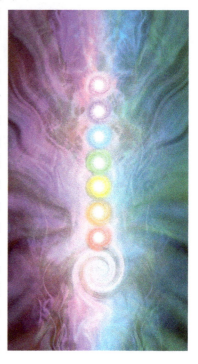

The technique which I used with David to re-energize the chakra energy centres involves imaging each colour of the rainbow on each of the different energetic points, from the base of the spine (tailbone) to the crown of the head. By imagining the colours and concentrating on breath, this becomes a relaxing, mindful experience. It is simple, short and easy to do. We found it very effective. I call it the rainbow visualization.

Let's Get Started

This visualization can be practiced anytime, either sitting comfortably or lying down. It could also be done at the end of your daily movement session for the added benefit of some extra relaxation ☺.

Find a quiet place where you will not be disturbed, maybe reduce the lighting so it feels more peaceful and calm. Make sure you are comfortable to begin your relaxation. This visualization may be done with or without soft music in the background.

You will find as each new colour builds in your mind a peaceful sense of calm and deep relaxation growing. There is no rush, take the time you want on each area before moving on to the next.

1.   Colour – Red.

Gently place your overlapped hands low down below your navel. This is your base or root chakra.

Close your eyes. Gently start with slow belly breaths, focusing your attention on the palms of your hands. Notice any sensations of warmth or cold in this area. As you start to relax you may start to feel some warmth generating in the palms of your hands.

Begin to imagine the colour red, a bright ball of red colour just beneath the palms. Sometimes it can help to repeat the word "red" as you inhale as it may help the mind to focus. With each exhalation release any tension and let it go. If you wish, you can also imagine the ball of colour spinning in a clockwise direction. Continue to focus on this area and establish a comfortable rhythm of breathing before moving on to the next colour.

Relax and breathe gently as you move from colour to colour.

2.   Colour – Orange.

Gently place your overlapped hands just below your belly button and focus on this area imagining the colour bright orange. This is your sacral chakra.

3.   Colour – Yellow.

Gently place your overlapped hands just above your belly button on stomach area. Focus on this area imagining the colour bright yellow. This is your solar plexus chakra.

4.   Colour – Green.

Gently place your overlapped hands over the centre of your chest. Focus on this area imagining the colour bright green. This is your heart chakra.

5.   Colour – Blue.

Gently place your overlapped hands over the base of your throat. Focus on this area imagining the colour bright blue / turquoise. This is your throat chakra.

6.   Colour – Indigo blue.

Gently place your overlapped hands over your brow in a relaxing position. Focus on this area imagining the colour indigo blue. This is your third eye chakra.

7.   Colour – Violet.

Gently place your overlapped hands at the top of your head. Focus on this area imagining the colour violet. This is the crown chakra.

When you have finished all areas, gently relax your hands, palms facing upwards, either by your side or in your lap. Take a quiet moment to enjoy the sensations from the relaxation, when you are ready, open your eyes.

Other forms of relaxation may include complementary therapies or participating in a relaxing activity.

Examples of some relaxing activities:

- Soaking in a bath
- Listening to soothing music.
- Being creative, painting, writing.
- Reading.
- Walking in nature.
- Stargazing.
- Yoga, Tai chi, Qigong.
- Sing and hum.

Research has shown that humming may ease stress, boost happiness and soothe sinuses.

Singing is known to release endorphins (feel good brain chemical that makes us feel happy and uplifted). There are also many other health benefits associated with singing and it's easy to make it a daily habit, even going up and down the notes of the scales in your shower daily or singing your heart out in the car counts!! Remember to smile when you're done. ☺

Holistic and Complementary Therapies

A complementary treatment is a natural type of treatment that is used alongside a conventional medical treatment. It may help you to feel better and cope better with your cancer treatment. An increasing number of doctors in the UK understand the benefits of complementary medicine for their patients and provide access, or referral, to some form of complementary therapy.

Benefits:

- Help reduce the side effects of cancer treatment.
- Help to reduce stress and anxiety.
- Help to improve physical and emotional wellbeing.
- Helps to feel more positive.
- Help improve recovery.

Although there are many complementary therapies widely available, some therapies can be safely integrated and others may be harmful depending on your individual circumstances. It is recommended to always check with your doctor before trying any of the treatments and take a doctor's note with you. Look for a recommended professional with experience of your condition and be sure they are fully aware of any medical treatment you may be receiving.

As a holistic therapist, over the years, I have found that the following treatments were particularly beneficial to my clients who have experienced cancer and could be integrated at different stages of their treatment. A diagnosis of prostate cancer and some of the prostate cancer treatments can cause side effects such as stress, anxiety and insomnia. These holistic therapies are intended to be soothing, relaxing and to help aid your wellbeing in general.

Massage Therapy

Massage therapy is used to help relax the muscles and reduce tension. Depending on the type of treatment you may be receiving for prostate cancer, it is possible that a massage may not be recommended for a certain period of time. Deep massage should be avoided and some massage techniques and the length of the treatment time may also need to be adapted whilst undergoing treatment. It is important to make sure you are hydrated both before and after your massage.

Reiki

I have found that Reiki is particularly helpful and soothing for those who are weak and fatigued. This is a non-invasive therapy, also known as energy healing that originated in Japan. It is used to help reduce stress, promote physical and emotional healing and encourage a healthy flow of energy. The client remains clothed and the practitioner places their hands lightly around or above the body, feet or head. Warmth can often be felt from the practitioner's hands during the treatment.

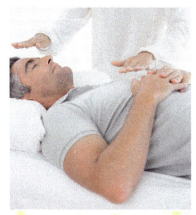

Reflexology

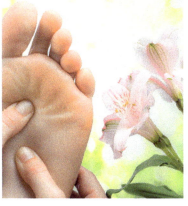

Reflexology is a deeply relaxing and energising holistic therapy. A gentle reflcxology treatment is non-invasive and comfortable to receive. A specific massage technique using thumb and finger pressure is applied to the reflex areas in the feet. The calming touch encourages the body to rebalance, decrease stress and anxiety and enhance sleep.

Diet and Hydration for Prostate Health

Diet plays an important role in health maintenance and resistance to illness. When we eat processed, preserved or devitalised foods, we weaken our system.

It is important where possible to eat good quality foods. Hormones and antibiotics injected into animals, pesticides sprayed on fruit and vegetables, air/water pollution, preservatives in food along with more recently genetically modified foods which have been introduced into the food chain, can have a profound effect on our long-term health.

The recommendation, where possible, is to eat natural foodstuffs which are in season and organic if possible.

Diet and supplements are a complex subject and particular to each individual, depending on their personal needs. In this section I have outlined some basic eating guidelines from a holistic perspective, where once again balance is the key.

Traditional Chinese medicine considers that the stomach is the engine which needs to be kept healthy to fuel the body and that cooked foods along with food and drinks at room temperature are beneficial, particularly when unwell, as they require less energy for digestion. When we have little energy, every little saving counts and can be directed towards healing instead.

Basics:

- Always have meals at regular times and eat healthy snacks.

- Give yourself time for proper digestion before retiring to bed.

- Watch portion sizes.

- Avoid alcohol and hydrate.

- Eat gut friendly foods.

The Gut Connection

It is considered holistically that the gut helps regulate your immune system.

The good bacteria which live in our gut is key in helping our immune system create a protective barrier against harmful bacteria and viruses. The good bacteria also help to provide a number of nutrients to our cells. Therefore, it is important to nourish your gut with gut friendly foods and consider the many factors which can influence and unbalance your gut health. e.g., Diet, antibiotics, toxins, stress, pollution, mouth hygiene and teeth.

The following list gives you some examples of gut friendly foods.

Polyphenols – They can reduce inflammation, play a role in brain function and memory. They are found in all plant foods, especially red and purple fruits such as red onions, tomatoes, wholegrains, pulses, beans, lentils and certain spices.

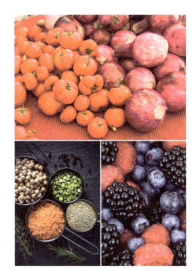

Fibre – Bacteria in the gut lives on fibre. By eating plenty of fruits, vegetables and wholegrains, you can provide your body with a variety of different fibres.

Fermented foods – Kefir, sauerkraut. Fermented proteins such as tempeh and natto.

Replace good bacteria – Studies show that it can be difficult to repopulate the gut with a good balance of bacteria following antibiotic use. This can be enhanced with prebiotic fibre and probiotic products.

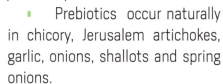

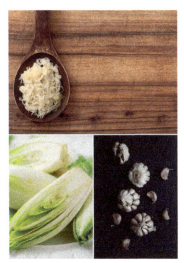

• Prebiotics occur naturally in chicory, Jerusalem artichokes, garlic, onions, shallots and spring onions.

• Probiotics contain live healthy bacteria and are found in fermented foods, miso, live culture yoghurts and kefir.

Healthy Foods

Below are some examples of healthy foods for prostate health.

- Fresh fruit and vegetables – 5 a day ☺
    - Fruit – 2 portions daily, particularly red and purple fruits.
    - Vegetables – 3 portions daily including cruciferous such as broccoli, cauliflower, cabbage, brussels sprouts, spinach, kale.
- Whole Grains – barley, brown rice, oatmeal, bulgur cracked wheat, millet.
- Pulses – in moderation. Soybeans, red kidney beans, pinto, chickpeas, lentils. (3 heaped tablespoons of pulses = 1 daily portion of veg).
- Seeds in moderation – 2tsp of flax seeds are considered beneficial when freshly ground daily. Pumpkin seeds daily or every other day.
- Nuts in moderation
- Soy foods – tofu, soy milk, soy yoghurts, soybeans. Avoid soy products with added salt and sugar.
- Seaweed
- Fish – wild caught ocean fish–salmon, tuna etc. At least 1 helping per week, more is better.

Foods to Avoid

- Processed foods with sugar.
- Processed meats – ham, bacon, sausages, burgers.
- White flour products
- Added salts.

- Fried foods.

- Dairy products – other than live culture yoghurt.

- Animal products –Avoid as much as possible. If animal products are eaten, use only organic products. Organic eggs are fine.

- Chemical additives.

- Fizzy drinks,drinks that contain caffeine e.g cola, coffee including decaffeinated, black tea.

- Beer and hard alcohol.

Hydration

Some treatments for prostate cancer can cause difficulty in urinating. Try to drink plenty of fluids 1.5/2litres a day (3-4pints). Caffeine products can irritate the bladder and make problems worse.

Avoidance of alcohol is recommended and is not helpful for hot flushes! However, if you do choose to have a drink, then no more than 1 glass of red wine a day.

In Traditional Chinese Medicine, it is also considered helpful to drink fluids at room temperature, or warm drinks, never chilled, especially when ill, as the body has to use not only energy for digestion but also to bring the drink to body temperature for optimum digestion.

Infusions:

- Green tea (decaffeinated variety)

- Sage tea – can possibly help with hot flushes.

- Chamomile tea

Proportions of Food:

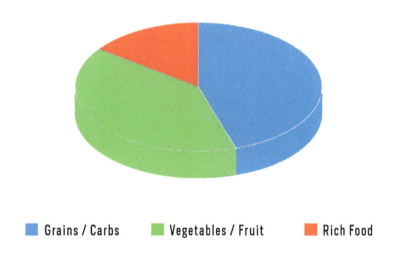

■ Grains / Carbs   ■ Vegetables / Fruit   ■ Rich Food

Basic guide

- 40–45% grains and carbohydrates.
- 35–40% vegetables and some fruit.
- 10–15% of rich foods such as seafood, free range eggs, fats, oils and sugars.

Supplements

Some supplements may interfere with your treatment for prostate cancer. It is important to check with your doctor first before taking any.

To Note:

A healthy balanced diet is imperative for the contribution towards overall good health by providing the fuel/energy needed to sustain healthy body functions.

- Don't eat or drink anything too cold as body loses energy in converting the extreme temperatures.

- Don't eat late before going to sleep: 3-hour rule for digestion.

- Book regular visits to your dentist to check gums and teeth and maintain good mouth hygiene, flossing etc. Bad bacteria in the mouth affects your digestive system and gut.

Summary

David continues today using the wellness practices which are outlined in this book. He has learnt, that even when you feel well, it is important to remember to do something every day in order to reap the constant benefits. Over time he has found that by incorporating the techniques regularly, they have now become a natural, integral part of his daily life for maintaining his wellness.

Below you will find a summary chart we created to highlight the different aspects of wellness which we covered within this book. For overall wellness it is important that none of the areas become neglected. You will also find a quick reference guide to help summarise the topics.

It's all about finding the balance and what you do every day that counts, even a small investment of time towards your wellness is always a something and so much better than a nothing. Remember, your body and mind will always thank you for it. ☺

Wellness Summary Chart

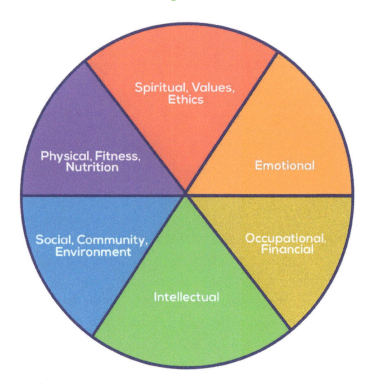

Emotional Wellness

- Good emotional health is important for maintaining a healthy immune system. Stress management helps with this and the use of mind/body relaxation techniques/ deep breathing exercises. Discover and use your personal stress reliever.

- *Calm your mind and body*. Your body responds to the way you think, feel, act. Use relaxation techniques to bring emotions back into balance. e.g. meditation, listening to music, listening to guided imagery tracks, practicing Yoga, Tai Chi, Qigong.

- Manage your time wisely because it will help lower stress.

- Find a balance between work and play, activity and rest.

- Have a regular routine for balance. Create healthy habits. Eat healthy meals, get enough sleep, exercise and stretch to relieve tension.

- Ask for help when needed.

- Find someone that you trust who you can openly share your feelings with.

- Seek professional help when you need it.

- Recognise when you are in an unhealthy relationship.

- Try recommended complementary therapies.

- Treat yourself.

- Spend time with positive people.

- Focus on the positive things in your life.

- Train your mind to think positive thoughts, practice mindfulness.

- Try to maintain a positive attitude even when problems arise.

- Accept change, keep things in perspective.

- Set yourself goals weekly, monthly to manage progress.

- Smile even when you don't feel like it.

Physical Wellness

- Take care of physical health. Exercise regularly, move body.

- Daily warm-ups.

- Balancing exercises.

- Kegels.

- Breathwork exercises.

- Yoga, Tai Chi, Qigong.

- Know when to stop, relax and rest.

- Find a balance between activity and rest. Balance energy out with energy in. Take time to restore, refresh, relax and rest.

- Get enough sleep. Try breathing exercises for insomnia, remember 3hr rule for digestion before going to bed. Avoid heavy meals, alcohol, caffeine, stimulants.

- Take care of your diet. Eat regular well-balanced meals. Watch portion sizes. Eat healthy, organic food where possible. Try to include 5 servings of fruits and vegetables in your diet every day. Avoid fried foods, white flour, soft drinks, processed meats and processed foods with sugar, dairy (except live culture yoghurt).

- Eat gut friendly foods.

- Hydrate. Avoid cold drinks.

- Avoid alcohol and toxic substances.

- Good mouth hygiene and regular dentist check-ups.

Spiritual Wellness

- Find a quiet place and spend time there every day.

- Chill out, relax, read.

- Contemplate the meaning of your life.

- Spend time appreciating the natural world around you. Spend time with nature.

- Be creative.

- Take time to explore your beliefs, values and ethics that help guide your life.

Social Wellness

- Have a strong social network with people who can give support and guidance when needed.

- Know who your best friends are.

- Balance your social life with family and friends.

- Connect with others, lunch date, coffee, pub, activities, join a group.

- Make sure your connections with others are positive

Financial wellness

- Take steps to live within financial means by financial planning and creating a budget.

- Be aware of the official benefits you are entitled to.

Intellectual Wellness

- Stay curious, engage in learning new things.

- Keep abreast of current affairs.

- Become a life-long learner.

Wellbeing Techniques – Quick Reference Guide

ACTION	BENEFIT
BREATHWORK	*Relieve stress and more*
Three part breath:	• Improve sleep quality/ Insomnia • Calm mind, soothe nervous system • Panic attacks • Relieve stress • Rejuvenate
Cooling breath:	• For hot flushes • When stressed / angry • When hot and overheated
Alternate nostril breathing:	• Calms mind • Refresh, reset • For mindfulness / relaxation
Four fold breath:	• Calm down fast
Abdominal breathing:	• Aches and pains • Afraid or tired
EXERCISES	*Help boost immune system, strength and mobility*
Daily warm ups:	• Circulation, relieve stiffness joints, muscles • Aids digestion
Balancing exercises:	• Core muscles • Calming, grounding

ACTION	BENEFIT
Qigong exercises:	• Improve energy/vitality
Kegel exercises: Yoga:	• Difficulty to urinate • Improve pelvic floor muscles • Maintain healthy prostate
DEEP RELAXATION TECHNIQUES	*Heal from stress*
Guided meditations:	• Rest/relax mind, balance emotions
Quick visualizations:	• Lift mood
Chakra rainbow visualization:	• Recharge/ rebalance
QUIET TIME	
Stop:	• Recharge, replenish
Relax:	• Energy in, rebalance
Sleep:	• Repair

Authors' Note:

We hope that this handbook / self help guide, for prostate health and a journey through prostate cancer will provide some light to all who read its pages.

Here is a little poem written for you.
Best wishes
David and Michelle

The Rainbow

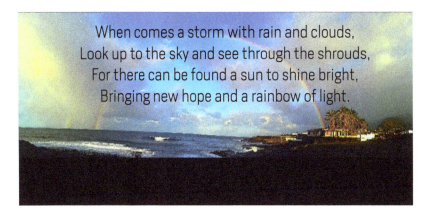

When comes a storm with rain and clouds,
Look up to the sky and see through the shrouds,
For there can be found a sun to shine bright,
Bringing new hope and a rainbow of light.

Information Contacts and Charities

Prostate Cancer UK   www.prostatecanceruk.org
Cancer Research UK   www.cancerresearchuk.org
Promotes testing   www.mypsatests.org.uk[**]
Promotes awareness   www.psatests.org.uk.[##]
Helpful information   www.prostatecanceruk.org
Reference   www.mholistictherapies.com
Reference/workshops   www.yoga-michelle.com
Contact   info@mholistictherapies.com

[**]   A charity funded and sponsored service which helps promote men aged 40 plus to get themselves booked on a local PSA testing event.

[##]   The Graham Fulford Charitable Trust promotes awareness of Prostate Cancer and offers home testing kits.

[*]   Donations to Rosemere Cancer Clinic and to Prostate Cancer Research. www.rosemere.org.uk

Acknowledgements

Special thanks to:

Theresa for your input and time given towards the production of this book.

Viv, Purple Parrot Publishing for your time, valuable contribution and publication.

Disclaimer

The information provided within this book is not intended as a substitute for the professional medical advice of physicians. The reader should consult a physician or general practitioner relating to his / her personal health before embarking upon recommendations within this publication.

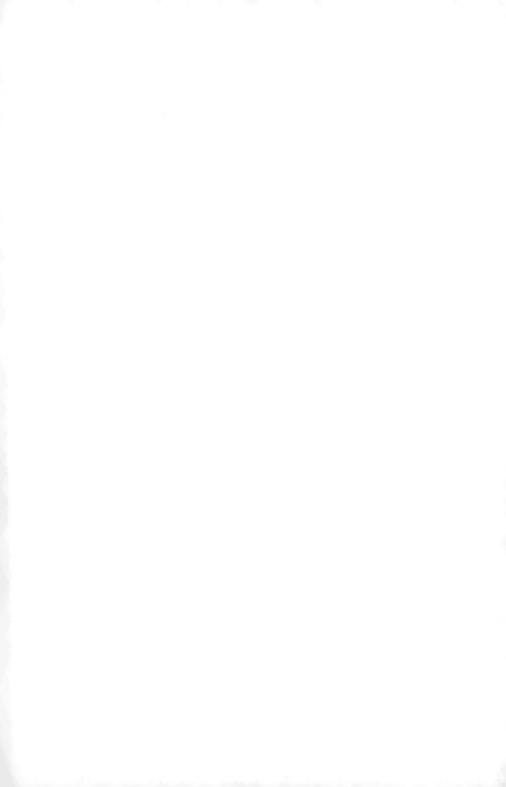